Making Medical Decisions

Making Medical Decisions

An Approach to Clinical Decision Making for Practicing Physicians

Richard Gross, MD, FACP

Professor of Medicine
University of Wisconsin Medical School
Madison, Wisconsin

American College of Physicians
Philadelphia, Pennsylvania

Acquisitions Editor: **Mary K. Ruff**
Manager, Book Publishing: **David Myers**
Administrator, Book Publishing: **Diane McCabe**
Production Supervisor: **Allan S. Kleinberg**
Production Editor: **Victoria Hoenigke**
Cover and Interior Design: **Patrick Whelan**

American College of Physicians (ACP) became an imprint of the American College of Physicians–American Society of Internal Medicine in July 1998.

Printed in the United States of America
Composition by ACP Graphic Services
Printing/binding by Versa Press

American College of Physicians–American Society of Internal Medicine
190 N. Independence Mall West
Philadelphia, PA 19106-1572

Gross, Richard, 1949–
    Making medical decisions: an approach to clinical decision making for practicing physicians / Richard Gross.
        p.   cm.
    Includes index.
    ISBN 0-943126-75-4
    1. Clinical medicine—Decision making—Handbooks, manuals, etc.
    2. Physicians—Decision making—Handbooks, manuals, etc.
    3. Evidence-based medicine—Handbooks, manuals, etc. I. Title.
    [DNLM: 1. Decision making. 2. Decision Support Techniques. WB
102G878m 1999]
    R723.5.G76 1999
    616—dc21
    DNLM/DLC
    for Library of Congress   98-29289
                                                                      CIP

99 00 01 02 03 04/9 8 7 6 5 4 3 2 1

To my late and dearly missed mother,
Annette Gross, whose devotion and love were
as certain as anything I have known

FOREWORD

If the long-running television comedy "Seinfeld" was a show about nothing, this book is a book about "not knowing."

Physicians are experts in "not knowing." We don't like it, we sometimes go to extremes to avoid it, but we cannot escape it. Alas, the nature of our chosen profession is that we always find innovative ways to generate uncertainty: new imaging techniques that show "lesions" that turn out to be inconsequential, new serum assays for ailments that turn out to be falsely positive as often as not. Uncertainty is a way of life for physicians, so why fight it? As I did with asparagus, get to know uncertainty, try a little at a time, and you may even get to like it.

Uncertainty is what this book is about (I think . . .). Before I began to comprehend the basics of decision analysis, uncertainty always created clouds of self-doubt and discomfort; it felt a little like ignorance. Now uncertainty is a comfortable companion. I know how to feel confident in my advice despite its presence, and I know that when I decide to fight uncertainty with increasingly aggressive tests or treatment choices, I am doing so because it will probably help my patient—not because it will simply make me feel more at ease.

So, even as medicine strives to reduce uncertainty through advances in science and conscientious continuing education, it will always be with us. I hope the concepts of this book will help you learn to feel as comfortable and self-assured with "not knowing" as you are with knowing.

CONTENTS

INTRODUCTION

꧁꧂

This book was written with a very specific goal: to teach key principles of medical decision analysis to clinicians so that they can use it in their practices. Like many tools born in academic settings, decision analysis has had only limited acceptance on the front lines, but it has such general applicability and is so well based on common sense that a special effort to transfer the "technology" from "gown to town" seemed worthwhile.

As a practicing physician who later became an academician, the author has been profoundly impressed by two seemingly paradoxical observations:

- Decision analysis offers profound insight and usefulness to practicing clinicians.

- Most practitioners do not use the discipline, at least not in an organized manner.

Unfortunately, within a short time after being introduced to decision analysis, most practitioners find that the cumbersome nature of its mathematics makes it difficult to incorporate into their routine.

It is the author's belief that what really counts is an understanding of the *logic* of decision analysis; it is at heart simple and elegant. The numbers and calculations are obviously important, but they can be easily dispensed with by a computer or mentally (using a few short-cuts). After all, how many of us resort to the Henderson-Hasselbalch equation every time we look at blood gas results? Similarly, in decision analysis we may rely on understanding the principles while letting the numbers sort themselves out in a routine manner.

It should be clarified that when the term *decision analysis* is used in this book, it is with considerable poetic license. What is actually discussed is a narrow but critical slice of decision science called *expected utility analysis*, or *threshold analysis*. This area of decision science was selected for its relevance, elegance, and intuitive "true-ness" for medical practice. There are many other aspects within decision analysis, including decision trees, complex statistical analyses, and sophisticated computer-based technologies, all of which are vital to specific purposes, but which are not needed for patient-based decisions in most cases. Therefore, the reader should be aware that when the term *decision analysis* is used in this book, we are referring to a specific aspect of the field.

HOW THIS MANUAL IS ORGANIZED

The sequence of this manual is as follows: First, we address some important conceptual issues relating to medical decision making.

Next, we present a few mathematical tools needed before entering the realm of decision analysis—namely, odds and probabilities. After that, we reverse the traditional sequence used in other texts (1) by first presenting *treatment* considerations (harm and improvement) and then presenting *testing* and diagnosis considerations (likelihood ratios, pre-test estimation). This reversal seems to make the learning process easier. The reason for the traditional sequence (testing concepts first, treatment concepts second) may be its mirroring of the usual course of patient care: test first, treat second. The reason for the sequence used in this book (treatment concepts first, testing concepts second) is that decisions about tests can be properly made only after a treatment's risks and benefits are analyzed. That is, understanding the risks and benefits of a treatment help one determine whether a test is worthwhile. So, with the material presented in this way, one can learn the concepts in a sequence that better reflects the way I hope that they will be used in practice. Finally, we discuss how to use all of these concepts together in order to make sound decisions at the bedside.

Several chapters in this manual are divided into two sections. The first section describes the principles, strategy, and logic in nonquantitative terms. Interested clinicians may confine their reading of these chapters to the first sections and still derive a meaningful appreciation of decision analysis. The second section of the divided chapters deals with the same material but in more quantitative terms. An attempt has been made to avoid overly technical and complex algebra. The reader should come away feeling that decision analysis is something he or she can actually use without further expertise.

To make this distinction easier to work with, the descriptive sections are printed in the same font as this Introduction. The quantitative sections are printed in the different font used in this sentence.

Numerous clinical examples are used in this book. The numbers they contain are generally clinically sensible. However, because the examples were designed to optimize clarity and process, the actual values may vary from those obtained through formal critical appraisal of the latest literature. In your use of decision analysis for patients, it is always desirable to apply rigorous standards of evidence.

This book is essentially a restatement of established ideas; it is lightly referenced, is written in an informal style, and has no pretensions about breaking new ground. Rather, the author hopes that some contribution is offered in the ways the ideas are presented, and in the fact that the vast gap that exists between academic decision science and front-line practice is narrowed a bit by this modest effort.

Chapter 1

DECISION ANALYSIS FOR PRACTICING PHYSICIANS: THE PROBLEM WITH PROOF

———∞∞∞———

Master clinicians often appear "intuitive" in their ability to make diagnoses and select treatments. Sometimes they do things that seem to defy traditional principles of scientific thinking. On the one hand, they may sniff out a rare diagnosis where others miss it; on the other hand, they may dismiss an esoteric diagnosis that others are advocating. Perhaps they exhibit great reluctance about a standard treatment, or they may proceed with a test or therapy even when the standard of care suggests waiting. Occasionally these sages are wrong, but often they are proved right.

Much remains to be learned about what is behind such feats of medical prowess, but we have learned that many master clinicians have acquired an intuitive grasp of the concepts we now call "heuristics" and "decision analysis." Fortunately, these are skills that any motivated clinician can acquire.

LIMITATIONS OF THE TRADITIONAL SCIENTIFIC METHOD IN CLINICAL PRACTICE

The scientific method has served us well and will continue to do so. It provides the "data" upon which we base our decisions. However, classic scientific thought in its application to clinical medicine has an important limitation: It demands absolute proof—unequivocal evidence—before a hypothesis is considered "accepted" (e.g., Koch's postulates). This concept of "proof" presents problems for clinicians because

1. Clinical diagnoses often cannot be truly "proved" other than by tests or procedures that are inherently impractical, dangerous, or inappropriate to the nature of the problem.

2. Tests are usually imperfect; they are almost never 100% sensitive or specific.

3. Varying patient preferences and desires cloud our concepts of any absolute "right" or "wrong," leading us (we hope) to adjust our decisions to reflect patient values.

4. Treatment, the end result of "proving" our clinical

hypotheses, invariably entails not only incomplete efficacy, but also costs and risks. It is not something we automatically advise simply because a diagnosis has been "proved."

As shown in Figure 1-1, attempts at truly "proving" something in clinical medicine are often an exercise in diminishing returns. Costs aside, you will learn that there is frequently no strategic value in increasing your clinical confidence beyond a specific, calculable level.

Thus, we usually fail to achieve certainty in medicine—*it is indeed a world dominated by uncertainty*. We can rarely hope to achieve anything close to the burden of proof imposed by clas-

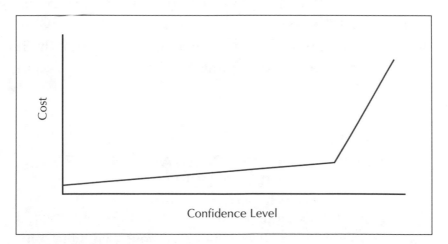

Figure 1-1. Typically, achieving reasonable diagnostic confidence requires a relatively small cost in time and resources. Moving from reasonable to very high levels of confidence may require disproportionate resources while contributing little to the decisions at hand. Much of decision analysis involves determining just how much confidence is "enough."

sic scientific theory when our "laboratory" is the examination room or the bedside. What we *can* do is approach the uncertainty in a scientific manner and avoid abandoning ourselves to vague speculation and anecdote; we need to approach uncertainty with confidence.

ENHANCING THE SCIENTIFIC METHOD

Decision analysis was conceived to identify the best choices under conditions of *likelihood* rather than certainty, and it incorporates not only quantitative measurements but also the subjective preferences of the individual patient. Those of us who have adopted these principles tend to find it difficult *not* to use them in our practices, and we can be an ornery lot because of this. It puzzles us why everyone doesn't think this way. In calmer moments, though, it becomes clear why the discipline has seen such slow acceptance by clinicians.

WHY ISN'T DECISION ANALYSIS MORE WIDELY USED?

One reason that decision analysis is not more widely used is that the concepts are a bit unfamiliar. Although no more difficult than many subjects that physicians have mastered for generations, decision analysis does not fit well into many classic medical paradigms. Interestingly, it sometimes leads to conclusions that seem counterintuitive, "unscientific," or "empiric" to physicians trained to acquire as much data as humanly possible before acting. It can be a bit disturbing to "act" or "not act" based on a decision analysis if one has been behaving otherwise for years.

WHY SHOULD WE USE DECISION ANALYSIS?

Decision analysis should be used for the same reason that you would bet on a royal flush but fold with a pair of two's; for the same reason you would wear seat belts or advise against smoking; for the same reason you would not advise buying a lottery ticket as a sound investment strategy. In short, decision analysis allows you to advise your patients about the "best bet." It can be a bit unsettling and even put you at odds with the "community standard" at times, but that is how standards come to change. If the decisions you make are in your patients' best interests, that is the only standard that matters.

In a book emphasizing probabilities and outcomes, it is with some embarrassment that I must acknowledge the lack of high-quality evidence about whether applying decision analysis (or evidence-based medicine in general) improves patient outcomes. On the other hand, the mechanics and mathematics are virtually axiomatic. Of course, the evidence on which decisions are based and the human values that color them will invariably leave questions behind. So, the *best* decisions may not always be *perfect* decisions but are always preferable to *random* decisions.

WHAT DECISION ANALYSIS IS *NOT*

As discussed in this manual, decision analysis is *not* a tool for making a differential diagnosis (although it can be helpful in deciding which tests are useful for confirming or excluding diagnoses). It will not help you generate a differential diagnosis. Support tools specifically designed for that purpose—such as QMR (First Databank, Inc., San Bruno, CA, 1996) and Iliad (Applied Medical Informatics, Salt Lake City, UT)—are far more helpful in that regard.

Having established a context for using decision analysis, we can now begin to explore the concepts behind it. Because most of the underlying principles of the discipline deal with the idea of "likelihood," this is the next topic to be addressed.

Chapter 2

LIKELIHOOD

⦿⦿⦿

PROBABILITY AND ODDS

Many definitions will be introduced in this text, but one concept seems to pervade virtually all areas of decision analysis and thus deserves its own chapter: **likelihood**.

Most readers will have little trouble grasping "likelihood" given the common usage of the word. It describes the statistical chance that an event will occur. In decision analysis, we generally express likelihood in one of two ways, **probability** and **odds**. In decision analysis, we use the related word *outcome* to describe a particular event; usually it is one of several possible events associated with a clinical situation, each having its own likelihood of occurring.

Example: If coronary bypass graft has a 1% chance of death, a 1% chance of stroke, and a 98% chance of success without either problem, each possibility (death, stroke, no complications) may be considered a separate *outcome* for that procedure.

PROBABILITY

Probability is the likelihood of the index outcome (that is, the outcome in question) expressed as a percentage of *all* outcomes. "All" includes the index outcome itself plus the other outcomes that may occur; thus, the index outcome is counted twice—once in the numerator and again in the denominator. For most of us, it is the most familiar way of expressing likelihood.

> **Example:** If we flip a coin 100 times, we may get 50 heads and 50 tails. The probability of heads is 50 out of 100, or 50%. The 100 figure includes the index outcome (heads) itself as well as the other outcomes that may occur (tails).

Probability looks at the entire universe of outcomes and compares any individual component outcome to this entire universe (including the original index outcome itself) as a percentage of the whole.

ODDS

Odds are less familiar to most of us. They are a means of expressing likelihood that compares the index outcome on the one hand and all *other* outcomes (*not* including the index outcome) on the other hand, to come up with a ratio of the two. They separate the index outcome from all other outcomes so that, unlike probability, odds count the index outcomes only once. In the coin toss analogy, odds would compare the 50 heads on the one hand with the 50 tails on the other hand for a ratio of 50:50, or 1.

Odds are like a seesaw with the index outcome on one side and all other outcomes (*not* including the index outcome) on the other (Fig. 2-1). The reason that odds are an important concept in decision analysis is that virtually all of the mathematical cal-

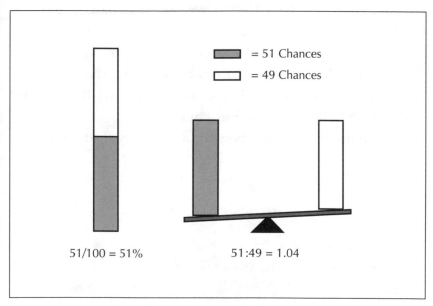

Figure 2-1. Two ways of expressing likelihood. *Left:* The likelihood shows the gray box as a proportion of the whole bar (probability). Right: The gray bar is "weighed" against the white bar, and the ratio of the two is calculated (odds).

culations one needs are either much simpler when expressed in their "odds form" or simply cannot be done using probabilities.

Why Use Odds at All?

If probability is so much more familiar, why bother with odds? The answer is apparent in the quantitative section of this chapter—the use of odds allows you to do quick calculations mentally that would be very difficult using probabilities because the formulas are too cumbersome. For this reason, it is important to develop an intuitive "feel" for odds.

Odds often "fit" better when you are making decisions. In most clinical situations, you face mutually exclusive possibilities. Knowing there are "two chances of this versus three chances of that" may lead to clearer thinking than knowing there is a "40% chance of this and a 60% chance of that." Either way is technically accurate, but patients are not often numerically experienced and whatever is conceptually clearer for them is best.

Getting a Feel for Odds

Odds Values are Asymmetric. Odds of 1 are equivalent to 50% probability, and any probability under 50% corresponds to odds somewhere between 0 and 1. Probabilities *over* 50% can go from odds just over 1 all the way up to infinity. Odds are thus not symmetric around the "midline" of 1. So, odds of 0.5 are not the same "distance" from 50% as odds of 1.5, even though both are "0.5 away from the midline" of 1. In fact, odds of 0.5 is the same as a probability of around 33%, and odds of 1.5 is the same as a probability of 60% (not 67%, which one might expect if there was symmetry) (Fig. 2-2).

Then again, odds of 99 are, coincidentally, roughly the same as 99%, so it is pointless to worry about odds much higher than that. When using odds intuitively, be careful that you take this into account.

Odds Know No Upper Limit. There are no odds that correspond to a probability of 100%; odds just get higher and higher without ever quite reaching complete certainty. So if you ever try to think in terms of odds and are faced with a likelihood that is certain or 100%, just use any very high number (such as 99 or 999) for odds and you will be close enough. You will see that

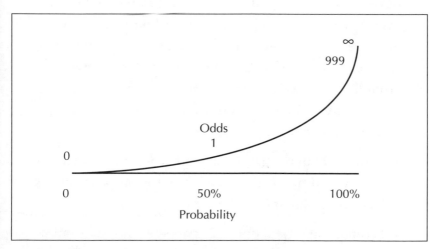

Figure 2-2. Odds are not symmetric around the "50-50" or break-even point. That is, all values to the left of "50-50" fall between 0 and 1, whereas values to the right of "50-50" range from 1 all the way to infinity.

trying to calculating odds equivalent to 100% probability results in infinity or in an obviously impossible division by zero.

Likelihood Must Be Taken in Context—Everything Is Relative

Likelihoods are powerful in clinical thinking because they reflect reality, but only to the extent that the context is well understood. By definition, likelihoods are relative to the "universe" from which they are calculated. The key is to knowing what "universe" you are dealing with.

Consider this:

> About 10% of all patients presenting with a *sore* throat have a true *strep* throat (2). You see a patient who clinically has approximately a 15% probability (odds = 0.18) of a strep throat based on suspicious physical findings, so you do a culture. Cultures are 90% sensitive and around 85% specific (there are many strep carriers who do not have disease). The throat culture is positive. Which of the following is/are correct?
>
> A. Because 9 out of 10 patients with a strep throat have a positive culture, you can be 90% sure that *your* patient has a strep throat (Fig. 2-3, *left*).
>
> B. Because roughly 13 out of 26 patients who have a positive culture actually have a strep throat, you can be 50% sure that *your* patient has a strep throat (Fig. 2-3, *right*).

In fact, sentence B is correct and sentence A is incorrect. The difference: the first half of each sentence refers to a specific "universe" of patients. Statement A is referring to the universe of *all patients with a strep throat* by some gold standard (e.g., increasing number of strep antibodies in the blood with an acute sore throat)—9 out of 10 patients *with a strep throat*. Because you do not know in advance whether *your* patient does or does not have a strep throat by that standard, you cannot use the 90% figure in thinking about your patient.

Statement B is referring to *patients like this one* (i.e., who have a positive culture). The likelihood that 13 out of 26 such patients will have strep is accurate and relevant.

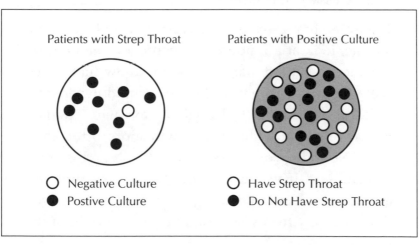

Patients with Strep Throat   Patients with Positive Culture

O   Negative Culture   O   Have Strep Throat
●   Postive Culture   ●   Do Not Have Strep Throat

Figure 2-3. Two patient populations. *Left circle.* Depiction of population of all patients with strep throat. Among these patients, there is a subgroup of patients with a positive culture. *Right circle.* Depiction of population of all patients with positive culture. Among these patients, there is a subgroup of patients with strep throat. The right circle best describes the patients that are of interest to us—those with a *positive culture*; the left circle, on the other hand, describes patients in whom a diagnosis has already been established.

The main point here is that any estimate of likelihood should always be associated in your mind with the universe from which it is drawn. You may wish to read this brief but tricky example again; consider to which populations the percentages given in each statement apply.

UNCERTAINTY

One of the advantages of thinking in terms of likelihood rather than certainty is that it never forces you to commit beyond what is either necessary or realistic.

> **Example:** In a game of "high card," two players ante a dime, look at a randomly drawn card, then decide whether to bet a dollar. You might know that a Jack will win most of the time, but you would never categorically state that "Jacks will always win." Rather, you would state, "Jacks will win more often than not." Nobody would cry foul if the Jack lost to a Queen. And if you bet on the Jack every time, on average you would make a good deal of money, even though at any turn you would never be certain of the outcome.
>
> Now, suppose instead that you reasoned that Jacks are good but that Aces are better. Therefore you will forfeit your Jacks each time (sacrificing the dime ante) without even knowing what your opponent has and wait to bet until you draw an Ace. You would pay a high price

indeed for the increased confidence that the Ace would bring you and, in fact, would end up losing in the end. True, you would feel mighty good about your certainty when the Ace did come up, but your wallet would be empty pretty quickly.

This analogy evokes what is often seen in clinical medicine. Think of a Jack as the likelihood of disease high enough to advise treatment. The Ace becomes an assessment that is more than adequate but at a much greater cost. We test and test and test to go from a Jack to an Ace, when the correct decision could have been made knowing it was a Jack all along. Poker players who always wait for a royal flush rarely win.

Here are three statements of good decision-makers who are comfortable with likelihoods:

"I am confident enough that the disease is present that I believe treatment is warranted."

"I believe that testing will provide us with the information we need to determine whether treatment is justified or not."

"I do not believe that testing is necessary because even a positive (negative) result would fail to change my mind about observing only (treating)."

LIKELIHOOD—QUANTITATIVE

PROBABILITY

In decision analysis, one uses a scale of probability that extends from 0 to 1 rather than from the usual 0% to 100%. A probability of 32% becomes 0.32, 5% becomes 0.05, and so on. Although we will continue to use percentages in the descriptive sections for their familiarity, whenever we revert to calculations, the 0-to-1 scale will be substituted.

ODDS

Odds make calculations much easier when you work with the formulas introduced in later chapters. Try to train yourself to switch easily between probability and odds. Remember that at higher likelihoods odds change greatly, whereas probabilities change little with the same variation in likelihood:

Probability	Odds
0.9	9
0.95	19
0.99	99

Here are the conversion formulas:

$$\text{Odds} = \frac{\text{Probability}}{1 - \text{Probability}}$$

$$\text{Probability} = \frac{\text{Odds}}{1 + \text{Odds}}$$

Chapter 3

TREATMENTS: HARM, IMPROVEMENT, AND BENEFIT

I t may seem that a book about decision analysis should save the chapter on treatments for the end. However, experience has shown that the subject of **treatment** is an ideal place to begin such a manual. Once the decision-oriented aspects of treatment are understood, the remaining principles become much more comprehensible. Treatment concepts may be a bit more challenging to grasp, but mastering these first makes it clear why one should care about the diagnostic testing concepts. The nontraditional order of presentation has thus proved superior in the author's teaching experience.

Although we treat in order to benefit those who have disease, we know that most treatments can cause harm; we hope to avoid treating those who do not have the disease. This chapter will discuss how to deal with these universal properties of treatment in a sensible way. Once you have mastered this topic, the remainder of the concepts should come readily.

OUTCOMES

Outcomes are simply well-defined events that occur as a result of either a disease or a treatment. Many diseases and treatments cause several possible outcomes. For example, treatment with oral penicillin in previously low-risk individuals causes rash (2%), diarrhea (2%), and anaphylaxis (0.0015%) (Drugdex System, Micromedex Health Care Series, Vol. 96, Micromedex, Inc., Englewood, CO, 1998); it also causes "no side effects" in most patients (95.9985%) (the numbers are illustrative only). Each of these is considered a separate outcome of treatment with penicillin. Similarly, diseases cause outcomes: streptococcal pharyngitis causes sore throat in 100% of patients, peritonsillar abscess in 5%, and so on. We will be concentrating on outcomes throughout much of the following discussion.

HARM, IMPROVEMENT, AND BENEFIT

Virtually every sensible treatment offers benefit to patients who have the disease for which it is intended. Penicillin reduces symptoms and mortality for patients with pneumococcal pneumonia, for example. Similarly, almost every treatment has the potential for harm; penicillin causes rash or diarrhea in a predictable percentage of patients (regardless of whether they have pneumonia).

Try to think of every disease–treatment scenario as having two possible components: how much *harm* the treatment causes in *healthy* patients, and how much disease *improvement* treatment brings about in sick patients.

Here is what this means (as with all examples used in this book, we are presuming "pure" situations—no other diagnoses or special circumstances should be imagined):

1. If you are certain that your patient does *not* have pneumonia but administer penicillin anyway, the patient could only stand to be harmed (albeit infrequently) and would have no possibility of benefit.

2. If the patient *does* have pneumococcal pneumonia and you administer penicillin, his or her fever, cough, and chest radiograph would improve and his or her rate of complications and risk of dying would decrease, on average, more so than if you did not administer penicillin. These outcomes improve with treatment.

3. Just like the healthy patient in the first example, the patient who does have pneumonia would be exposed to penicillin side effects. When you factor in these side effects, a net benefit would persist, although it would be a bit less than it would be if there were no side effects.

These three examples describe, respectively, the essence of the concepts **harm, improvement, and benefit** as they relate to decision analysis.

A more general description of these concepts is as follows:

Harm: the adverse consequences of a treatment that would occur in a patient *without* disease ("side effects in healthy persons").

Improvement: how much better the patient with *disease* does *with* treatment compared with what his or her condition would be without treatment, disregarding the side effects of the treatment ("patient betterment").

Benefit: how much better the patient with disease does with treatment compared with what his or her condition would be without treatment, after *accounting for the side effects* of the treatment ("patient betterment less the side-effects").

The term *improvement* is not traditional in this context (I hope for good didactic reasons), so new learners should be aware that previous works may use alternative definitions. *

---

*Note to experienced decision analysts: We have the possibility of confusion here. The term *benefit* is sometimes used to mean *improvement* (as defined above), whereas the term *net benefit* is used to mean *benefit minus harm*. Some works (1) do not use the term *net benefit* at all, but rather use *benefit* to mean *net benefit*. (To add to the confusion, Sox and colleagues also do not use the term *harm*, but rather use *cost* to mean the same thing, although the literal cost is also referred to as such in cost–benefit calculations.) The author has seen otherwise superb curricula use the term *benefit* in one section, and then use *net benefit* in others, all the while meaning *net benefit* in both cases. It is a daunting task for the new learner to sort this out.

Using the terms *harm, improvement,* and *benefit*, I have found it much easier to teach the concepts that follow. It allows direct use of the probability form of the action threshold (as shown below), obviating yet another odds-to-probability calculation; it makes it unnecessary to distinguish benefit from "net" benefit, substituting a neutral term ("improvement") for clarity; it conceptually separates the treatment's side effects from its "helpfulness" as two mutually independent ideas.

SANITY CHECKPOINT

Regarding the definition of *harm* we have just discussed, you may be wondering why on earth anyone would take a treatment for a disease they didn't have. Well, they wouldn't— if they *knew* that they didn't have disease. The problem is that they may end up taking the treatment on their physician's advice even when they don't have the disease. For example, a clinician may prescribe antibiotics after making a diagnosis of pneumonia based on cough, a few crackles on lung examination, and fever—when, in fact, the patient does not have pneumonia, only a cold. Or a clinician may obtain a chest x-ray and misinterpret an incidental old lung scar as a sign of acute pneumonia. Because *harm* refers to treated patients without disease who receive treatment, these two patients qualify for the *harm* definition. The inadvertent treatment of the healthy patient may be "good medicine" in its intent and by community standards, but there will be those instances in which it is incorrect.

Consider the above definitions of *harm, improvement,* and *benefit* in the following example:

> **Example:** Gorillatoxan (a fictional agent) given to patients with pancreatic cancer reduces the 12-month mortality due to the cancer from 50% to 20%. That is, it results in 30 fewer deaths from the cancer at 12 months for every 100 patients treated. Unhappily, it also causes fatal brain hemorrhages in 10% of patients who take it. That is, it kills 10 patients for each 100 patients treated. In this case, the **improvement** is 30 fewer deaths, the **harm** is 10 drug-related deaths, and the final **benefit** is 30 – 10, or 20 fewer deaths.

The concepts will become important in the next chapter on action thresholds.

MEASURING HARM AND IMPROVEMENT: PATIENT "UTILITIES"

In defining harm and improvement, we use general phrases such as "how much the patient's condition improves" and "how bad are the side effects of treatment." However, in actual decision making about a specific patient, these ideas need to be expressed more precisely and objectively.

First, we must recognize that one person's judgment of a "good" or "bad" clinical outcome may be quite different from that of another person. For this reason, virtually every clinical decision must take into account *the preferences and values of the individual patient.*

> **Example:** A sedentary accountant is faced with the possibility of losing her first toe as a risk of a proposed surgery. She hardly likes this prospect, but could continue her life after such a loss with minimal impact on overall income, leisure activities, and other quality issues. She judges this outcome to be a mild-to-moderate side effect.
>
> Her identical twin sister has chosen to be a ballet dancer, at which she is quite successful, and she is trained or inclined to do little else. Faced with the same prospects, she judges loss of her toe to be a severe side effect.

Although we can help our patients to make sensible judgments by elucidating facts and consequences, there is clearly no "right" or "wrong" value in most cases—the patient is the final judge. We can also help our patients be consistent in their value judgments. The term used to describe the personal judgment of "goodness" or "badness" that a patient places on a particular outcome is **utility**. Usually, perfect health is the best outcome, and death and similar horrible outcomes are the worst.

Utility is a measure of the relative "goodness" or "badness" of a disease or treatment outcome, relative to the other outcomes that may occur in the scenario under consideration. The "score" is assigned by the patient as a value judgment, generally expressed as an absolute, unitless number from 0 to 1 (bad to good). Although other systems exist for expressing utilities (e.g., quality adjusted life years, or QALYs), for purposes of clarity we will stick to the simpler 0-to-1 scale. In this context, lower is always worse and higher is always better.

Utility represents the *subjective* dimension of an outcome. The other dimension of the outcome is the *likelihood* of the outcome. A very bad outcome (that is, one with a very low "utility" for the patient) may occur in only one patient in 200,000 (e.g., anaphylaxis caused by penicillin). In this case, although the utility is very low (i.e., very bad), its likelihood is also very low, making it overall a fairly minor factor in our decision. Few would hesitate to take the usual oral antibiotics for an appropriate indication; there is a definite risk of death from doing so, but at a rate of one per 200,000, we discount it by virtue of its rarity.

Thus, one must consider both utility and likelihood when judging the importance of an outcome in the decision making process. It is the *product* of the two that is used in formal analyses.

IMPACT

In subsequent chapters, we will make use of a related concept: **impact** (like the term *improvement*, *impact* is new to the terminology of decision analysis). Impact is similar to utility, but instead of being measurable on a bad-to-good scale, it is simply a reflection of how much an outcome affects the patient relative to his or her not experiencing the outcome at all, regardless of the "goodness" or "badness" of the outcome. With utility, lower is always worse and higher is always better. With impact, the only issue that counts is *how profoundly an outcome affects the patient* (much like the popular "stress scales," in which both a happy wedding and the death of a loved one cause substantial "stress" despite one being pleasant and the other not). *

---

*Note to experienced decision analysts: The introduction of impacts is a tool for the teaching of expected utility analysis. Theoretically it is similar to utility; however, by maintaining a unidirectional numeric assignment about the importance of an outcome (rather than a scale such as that used in measuring utilities, where harm is lower and benefit is higher), impacts can be applied to both the denominator and numerator of the action threshold equation. Without this, one must resort to the traditional $(U[D-T-] - U[D-T+])/(U[D+T+] - U[D+T-])$ approach, which few new learners will tolerate for long. Its disadvantage is that there is a risk of oversimplification in more complex scenarios. Combined with the use of improvement instead of benefit (thereby allowing direct use of the probability form of the action threshold equation as shown elsewhere), this approach has proved remarkably successful in my teaching experience; its finer points can be filled in after the learner achieves confidence about the basic concepts.

Another subtle but important difference between impact and utility: utility refers to the score of a given health outcome as an independent state. Impact reflects the implied *difference* between living *without* the outcome compared with living *with* the outcome. Utility is assigned to a health state regardless of how much it differs from another health state (the differences are calculated later in the decision making process).

A severe side effect would have a strong "impact" on a patient, as would a dramatic cure from a serious disease. Both could have an impact of 0.9 on a 0-to-1 scale. Simply think of impact as an "importance score" for health outcomes (Fig. 3-1).

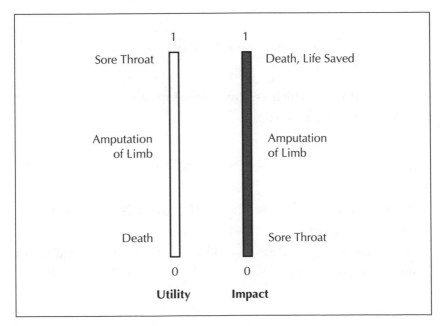

Figure 3-1. *Utility* and *impact* both measure a patient's judgment of a health outcome. **Utility** does so on a "bad-to-good" scale, from 0 to 1. With **impact**, only the importance of an outcome is considered; the "goodness" and "badness" of the outcome is not considered.

Impact and utility ultimately give the same results in the final decision calculations. You will see shortly that impact allows quick estimates of important decision parameters, whereas utility requires more math; you will also see that in complicated situations, one must use utility, after all.

SUMMARY

In summary, harm and improvement can be defined in terms of

1. The good effects of treatment manifested as betterment of the patient.

2. The bad effects of treatment, which we generally call *side effects* or *risks*.

3. The impact, which is how important a patient perceives a given outcome to be.

Harm is the likelihood of the side effect multiplied by its **impact**.

Improvement is the likelihood of patient betterment multiplied by its **impact**.

Armed with these ideas, we will discuss in the next chapter how to put them to use.

HARM, IMPROVEMENT, AND BENEFIT—QUANTITATIVE

THE SIMPLIFIED METHOD

There are two ways of approaching the quantitative aspects of harm and improvement: the **simplified** and **advanced** methods. The simplified method is highly intuitive and can be readily used at the bedside. I believe it is extremely useful in making the best decisions for our patients, although there is actually no established way of testing its validity. That is, the logic behind it is mathematically solid, but there are no randomized, controlled trials to confirm its "efficacy." On the other hand, all methods of assessing harm and improvement rely on subjective estimates of utilities, so there probably is no "correct" decision except as it applies to an individual patient. Here is how it works:

Harm is estimated by first determining the *likelihood* that a side effect will occur if the treatment is given to a healthy patient (use probability [0 to 1] rather than odds). It is acceptable to combine into a single probability two or more side effects if they have similar "impacts" (in more complex situations, the advanced method discussed on p 33 below is more appropriate). Next, assume that a healthy patient did, in fact, experience these side effects and that the patient assigned a number from 0 to 1 to the *impact* the side effects would have on his or her life. Assume that 1 is the highest score (i.e., the most important impact imaginable, such as death) and 0 is the lowest score (i.e., virtually no impact). Finally, multiply the impact by the likelihood:

$$Harm = Probability \times Impact$$

Next, repeat the above procedure for *improvement*. How likely is a patient *with* disease to derive "betterment" from the treatment? And how strong is the *impact* of that betterment? Ignore side effects from treatment when making this estimate. In this case, an impact of 1 means tremendous betterment (such as a life saved), and low numbers mean virtually no betterment. As with harm:

$$\text{Improvement} = \text{Probability} \times \text{Impact}$$

Example: Penicillin causes rash and diarrhea in 4% of patients for approximately 5 days. It relieves strep throat symptoms by reducing pain from 6 days to 4 days—that is, by 2 days. For **harm**, I would estimate the impact of rash and diarrhea to be quite low—say, 0.01 on the 0-to-1 scale.

So,

$$\text{Harm} = 0.04 \times 0.01, \text{ or } \mathbf{0.0004}$$

Improvement accrues to virtually all patients with strep throat, so probability is essentially 1. I estimate the impact to be minimal (2 fewer days of having a sore throat)—say, about one third as much as the 5-day rash/diarrhea impact discussed above. Because I assigned that a score of 0.01, I will give this impact a score that is about one third of that: 0.003.

So,

$$\text{Improvement} = 1 \times 0.003 = \mathbf{0.003}$$

The exact numbers you choose for the impact values are not critical; it is their *relative size* that matters. In the above example, I assigned the impact for harm a score of 0.01 and that for improvement a score of 0.003. Had I chosen to give harm a 0.9 and improvement a 0.3, the ratio would be the same (3:1) and the results would be the same! If you fret that your impact estimates are too arbitrary, stop worrying. Worry instead about whether the impacts for harm and improvement are in *correct proportion* to each other.

You will see in the next chapter how these numbers can be put to great use in calculating the action threshold.

THE ADVANCED METHOD

Author's Warning: New learners are advised to skip this section and complete the rest of the book. You may return here after a good meal at a later time. Reading it now may well break your train of thought and disrupt the continuity of the chapters.

I don't think I would attempt the advanced method if I were a busy practitioner without academic time. (I say this reluctantly because I know that it is the "gold standard" and some of my colleagues might be very cross with me.) Experience has shown the advanced method to be too cumbersome for routine "front line" use, at least without a computer program to help,* and the simplified method is usually adequate for the clinician at the bedside.

Still, for the curious or those interested in understanding the entire process, it is presented below.

In any clinical scenario, a patient either has the index disease or does not; also, the patient either receives treatment or does not. Thus, one can describe a patient as falling into one of four "disease-treatment" **states**, where D is disease and T is treatment, and + means present and – means absent:

1. **No disease, no treatment**—designated **[D–T–]** (e.g., a healthy patient: the test was negative and no treatment given)

2. **No disease, but treated**—designated **[D–T+]** (e.g., the patient had a viral sore throat, but a false-positive strep screen led the physician to prescribe antibiotic treatment)

3. **Disease without treatment**—designated **[D+T–]** (e.g., the patient had a strep throat but a false-negative strep screen and therefore did not receive treatment)

4. **Disease plus treatment, net results**—designated **[D+T+]** (e.g., the patient had strep throat and a positive strep screen; treatment was given and side effects were account-ed for)

The first and last states (states 1 and 4) are what we aim for but are not always what we attain. Note that each state describes a unique "disease/no disease" and "treatment/no treatment" status.

---

*Such computer tools are available and should not be disregarded if you think that you are likely to become enthusiastic about decision analysis. Later in the text (p 74) I present a simple spreadsheet template you may try for starters. There are Internet sites of relevance, including one by the author: www.decisions.medicine.wisc.edu (accurate at the time of this printing, although, as with all things digital, this information may change). Finally, a robust decision analysis and evidence database program is discussed in Appendix D.

Next, we examine each of these states by listing all of its possible outcomes in a table. For each outcome, we list the probability and utility as shown below; then we multiply the utility by the probability to obtain the rightmost column, labeled "U × P." Finally, we sum the results of all the U × P columns to derive a number we call the **"expected utility"** for that health state.

Consider the expected utility for *untreated disease* (U[D+T−]). A table like this could be created for high-grade carotid stenosis:

Outcome	Probability	Utility	U × P
Death	0.1	0	0
Stroke	0.05	0.3	0.015
Cure	0.85	1	0.85
Total	**1.00**		**0.865**

The sum of the *probabilities* of all rows must equal 1. In addition, the individual outcomes must not overlap in terms of which patients they include: they should be mutually exclusive (not always an easy task). This means that in the case of treatments, one usually needs to add an outcome such as "No side effects" to allow the sum of all probabilities to equal 1.

In this example, we had no treatment outcomes to consider, but if we did, we would simply add them to the list of possible outcomes in the same manner. Some or all of the disease outcomes would presumably be different from what they are without treatment, and the list would contain additional outcomes that reflect side effects of treatment.

An Aside for Obsessive-Compulsives: One weakness of this model is that it is easy to imagine patients deriving betterment from the treatment but also having an unrelated side effect. If the side effect happens to be an outcome that is the same as one of the disease outcomes, it can be easily factored in. If it is an outcome that the disease cannot cause, a dilemma occurs: Outcomes are supposed to be mutually exclusive, yet some patients will obtain both betterment and this unrelated side effect. This situation is not gracefully handled using this model; often we "steal" the side effect group from the group of patients who derive no betterment from treatment in order to "force" the total probabilities to equal 1. This technique can thus get confusing for complex scenarios. For this reason, alternative approaches such as decision trees are superior in such cases (3,4). Although beyond the scope of this discussion, clinical scenarios requiring that level of sophistication seem uncommon in everyday practice. Decision trees are discussed in Chapter 8.

The **expected utility** of this state is the sum of the right-hand column (0.865 in this case).

With this vocabulary, we can quantitatively redefine *harm*, *improvement*, and *benefit*:

Harm is the expected utility for perfect health (i.e., no disease, no treatment, U[D-T-]), minus the expected utility for "no disease, treatment only," or U[D-T+].

$$U[D-T-] - U[D-T+]$$

The left-hand part of this equation (U[D-T-])is usually assumed to be 1, because it is normal health: no disease, no treatment.

Benefit is the expected utility of disease with treatment including its side effects, minus that of disease without treatment:

$$U[D+T+] - U[D+T-]$$

Improvement is the expected utility for treated disease (but this time ignoring the treatment side effects) minus the expected utility for untreated disease. This represents how much better the disease does with treatment than without.

$$U[D^{Rx}] - U[D+T-]$$

The key element here is $U[D^{Rx}]$, the state for which you consider the disease behavior that occurs with treatment while disregarding the treatment side effects themselves.

> **One caveat:** When constructing the tables described above, you should keep your utility scores "global" across the tables. That is, do not use 0 and 1 as the best and worst outcomes for each table. Rather, use 1 as the score for the best outcome for all of the rows in *all* of the tables, and 0 for the worst outcome for all of the tables. Within any given table, therefore, your best "row" may have a score of 0.85 if there is a better row in one of the other tables.

The next section offers guidance in determining how to assign utilities to the outcomes that fall between the best and the worst—intermediate utilities.

INTERMEDIATE UTILITIES

It is relatively easy to identify the best and worst outcomes across a scenario as described previously, with these outcomes receiving a 1 and 0, respectively. Determining utilities for outcomes that fall *in between*, however, is less straightforward.

Normal health and death might be the two extremes, but what about assessing "losing a leg" or "left-sided paralysis?" A technique often used for this purpose is called the **standard gamble**. It works like this:

1. For the utility in question, create a two-choice dilemma: You have before you two doors. If you choose door 1, you are 100% certain to experience [intermediate outcome] (Fig. 3-2). If you choose door 2, you will have a 50% chance of experiencing [best outcome] and a 50% chance of experiencing [worst outcome]. Which door would you choose?

2. Each time the patient selects a door, adjust the original 50%/50% gamble for door 2 to make the choice more difficult. That is, if they opt for the "sure thing" (door 1), make the "gamble" (door 2) a little more attractive: "If you choose door 2, you will have a 75% chance of experiencing [best outcome] and a 25% chance of experiencing [worst outcome]." Use your judgment in selecting the actual amount of change you apply each time, but the idea is to repeatedly bracket the patient's choices.

3. Sooner or later, the choice will become virtually impossible to make. In other words, it will be a toss-up.

At this stage, the probability for the *best* outcome from door 2 at the time of the "*toss-up*" becomes your new intermediate utility. By practicing this technique a few times, you will be able to help patients quickly arrive at a consistent utility for all of the outcomes in your scenario. Not all patients will grasp the concepts, but for those who do it is quite useful.

Other methods exist for accomplishing this goal, such as the "time trade-off" method. This involves asking a question such as

How many years living in good health would you accept in return for living 10 years with paralysis of your left side and inability to speak?

Or, more generically:

How many years living in [best state] would you accept in return for living 10 years with [intermediate state]?

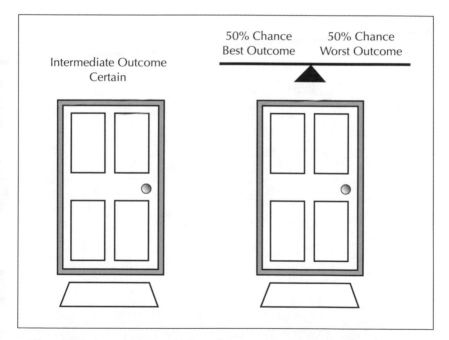

Figure 3-2. The patient is asked which door he or she would prefer. Sequentially, the 50%/50% figure shown for the door on the right is adjusted to make the choice more difficult until it is a "toss-up." The toss-up figure for the best outcome for the door on the right reflects the intermediate utility being estimated.

The intermediate utility is the patient's reply as a proportion of 10 (or whatever time span you choose to make the question plausible).

Sox and colleagues provide further information on both the "standard gamble" and "time trade-off" methods (1).

Chapter 4

TREATMENTS: ACTION THRESHOLD

———∞∞∞———

T he decision analyst's concept of harm and improvement was addressed in previous chapters. We will now build on this to explain one of the most important ideas in clinical decision making: the **action threshold**.

BALANCING HARM AND IMPROVEMENT

Let us think of two treatment scenarios in a traditional, intuitive manner:

1. Dangerous treatments such as chemotherapy for cancer may cause great harm and offer only a small benefit even if you are certain that the disease is present: The *improve-*

ments that they offer may be only a little better than the harmful side-effects. If there were even a small doubt about whether the disease was present, the overall risks of treatment would not be worth taking. Your *confidence in the diagnosis* would have to be very high before you would recommend taking action. Perhaps you would want to be 98% sure that you were right. Biopsy and similar tests would be routinely recommended.

2. On the other hand, benign treatments such as oral antibiotics for outpatient pneumonia may offer little risk of harm and great likelihood of improvement. It may be that if there were even a relatively small possibility of pneumonia, the treatment risks would be worth taking. Although you would never treat without some basis for the diagnosis, your threshold of confidence for recommending action may be relatively low—say, 50%. To be on the safe side, you might just go ahead and treat a moderately ill patient even if the radiographic abnormalities were equivocal, rather than observing or ordering expensive but nonspecific sputum cultures, blood cultures, CT scans, and so forth.

What we are describing here is the concept of the **action threshold**. In considering these two scenarios, your thoughts may have gone something like this:

"In the chemotherapy patient, the risks of treatment are very great, and I would be quite upset if I exposed even a small number of healthy patients to this risky treatment. Although patients with cancer would also risk getting side effects, at least they would stand a chance of deriving enough overall improvement for their trouble to justify this risk. I would need a very high level of confidence in the diagnosis before I would advise treatment."

"For the pneumonia patient, it is true that I am not actually that certain that pneumonia is present, but it might be. If I fail to treat pneumonia, its morbidity and mortality will be much higher than if I treat it. It is no big deal if I inadvertently treat some patients who do not have pneumonia, because the treatment is not that bad. All in all, treatment is the safest route to go. I really need only a moderate level of confidence in the diagnosis before I would advise treatment."

Your **action threshold** for both of these cases reflects just how confident about the diagnosis you needed to be before advising treatment; it was high in the first case, moderate in the second case. It is a way of expressing the risk-to-improvement index of a treatment in terms of the diagnostic confidence it requires in order to be the best decision.

The action threshold is a property of a *treatment* for a specific *disease*. It is the likelihood of disease above which the treatment will, on average, provide more improvement than harm, and below which the treatment will cause more harm than improvement.

One might say that above the action threshold, treatment is your "best bet."

The above definition is a pivotal concept. You will soon see how to determine the action threshold in a less subjective way.

Here are important corollaries of this definition:

- If your likelihood of disease is *lower than* the action threshold, you should not treat.

- If your likelihood of disease is *higher than* the action threshold for its treatment, you should treat.

- If a given test would change your diagnostic confidence from one side of the action threshold to the other, it has high decision value; if not, it has low decision value.

It is worthwhile remembering that we are "playing the odds." Some patients whose disease likelihood falls below the action threshold will do better with treatment, and some whose disease likelihood lies far above it will end up worse off by taking treatment. Still, given the inherent uncertainties, the odds favor benefit for those whose disease likelihood is above the action threshold and harm for those whose likelihood is below the action threshold.

Such is the essence of making a treatment decision. There are no guarantees about individual results, but because we have accounted for the known outcomes of the disease, the treatment, and the patient's values, we have done everything we can to stack the deck in favor of a correct decision. You may not win every bet by doing this, but in the end, the patient usually comes out ahead.

A *decision* to treat is correct regardless of whether the disease likelihood is only a little bit above the action threshold or whether it is far above the action threshold. The difference is that the former patient is only a little more likely to derive benefit from treatment, whereas the latter patient is highly likely to derive benefit. Both patients are better off receiving treatment.

Now for the easy part: To calculate the action threshold as a probability, simply divide the *harm* by the *improvement* (as derived in the previous chapter):

$$\text{Action Threshold} = \text{Harm}/\text{Improvement}$$

If you wish to stick with the **odds form**, use the following calculation:*

$$\text{AT\_Odds} = \text{Harm}/(\text{Improvement} - \text{Harm})$$

Either form (probability or odds) gives you the likelihood of disease you would need in order to be certain that treatment is the best decision.

---

*Some medical articles leave you little choice but to use the odds form. This is because they do not report the treatment side effects (*harm*) as a separate number, especially when these side effects are the same as one or more of the possible disease outcomes, such as death. For example, they report mortality rates in two cohorts, one with and the other without treatment; although the treated group may have a lower mortality, we sometimes cannot know whether the improvement is owing to small disease improvement teamed with minimal mortality with treatment, or to a larger disease improvement offset by a greater mortality with treatment. When all you can glean are the final outcomes with and without treatment, you should generally use the odds form of the action threshold (*harm/benefit*), not the probability form (*harm/improvement*). The benefit is then the difference between the two cohorts, and the harm is whatever side effects are reported separately in the article. This may take the form of *undesirable* outcomes that occur *more* frequently in the treated cohort, even if not explicitly labeled as a side effect or harm. When using the odds form, remember to convert the action threshold back to probability, as discussed in earlier chapters.

I find it much more informative when I can "tease out" the role of side effects from the overall effects of the treatment. Compare two disease–treatment scenarios: one in which the mortality with disease improves from 50% to 10% but in which the treatment causes death in 39% for a benefit of 1% decrease in mortality, compared with another in which the mortality with disease improves from 50% to 49% and the treatment is virtually harmless. The net effect is the same, but somehow the patient's decision (or the clinician's) may vary, depending on his or her personal feelings about dying from a disease compared with dying from a side effect of its treatment. Inquiring minds may want to know . . .

Note: We have assumed that, for patients with disease, the probability of side effects is the same as that for healthy patients, which is usually true. However, sometimes in patients with disease there is a higher incidence of side effects than in healthy persons. For example, the incidence of heart attack due to catheterization is higher in patients with severe coronary disease than in those without the disease; ampicillin rash occurs more frequently in patients with infectious mononucleosis than in those without the disease (0.09 vs. 0.5) (Drugdex System, Micromedex Health Care Series, Vol. 96, Micromedex, Inc., Englewood, CO, 1998), and so on. There are advanced ways of dealing with this when necessary, but for our purposes, just be aware that this occasionally comes up and can alter the conclusions: You would be more likely either to treat or to observe and less likely to use the test to help you decide.

GOING AGAINST THE GRAIN

Given these principles, you do not need to be sure about a diagnosis in order to make a proper recommendation of treatment or observation. You need to know only whether the likelihood of disease is above or below the action threshold. **That is, you can be *certain* about the best advice even when you are *uncertain* about the diagnosis and ultimate outcomes.**

PLAYING THE ODDS

We used the analogy of the card game when discussing likelihoods. Action thresholds also have gambling analogies that are helpful:

Example: Consider a lottery using black and white marbles in a basket, where drawing a black marble is a "win" (Fig. 4-1). If we have determined that the basket contains 51 black marbles and 49 white ones, we would always bet on black, although we would not always win. The same advice would hold if the basket contained 90 black ones and 10 white ones. We do not need to know anything beyond "51:49" in order to advise a player to bet on black rather than white. Whatever effort or cost is necessary to discover whether it was 51:49 versus 90:10 is useless in terms of whether to bet on black or white.

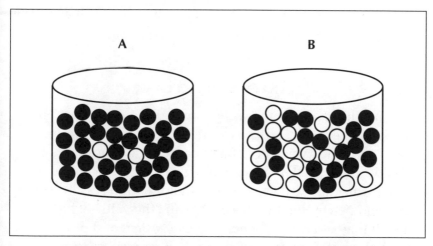

Figure 4-1. Basket A has a 33:2 black-to-white ratio. Basket B has a 20:15 black-to-white ratio. If forced to "bet" on which color is more likely to be randomly drawn from each basket, a numerate bettor would choose black in both cases—the "threshold for betting on black" is 50% because anything higher would win more often than it would lose. In terms of which way to bet, there is no value in knowing whether the ratio is 33:2 or 20:15. Similarly, once a diagnosis likelihood exceeds the action threshold, there is no "decision value" in increasing your diagnostic confidence.

The action threshold works the same way. Once we have finally determined that the disease likelihood is above the action threshold, the correct "bet" is to treat; below the action threshold the best bet is not to treat.

ISN'T IT BETTER TO BE AS CONFIDENT AS REASONABLY POSSIBLE?

Assuming you are obliged to bet (as are all patients with a disease—namely, whether to take treatment or not), you may well ask how much it is worth to learn that the odds are 90:10 instead of 51:49 when deciding on which is the best bet? The answer is that it is worth little or nothing in most cases.

SANITY CHECKPOINT

You may have a gnawing feeling that, although we can probably give the correct advice about treating or observing based on being even a little bit over the action threshold, it would still be "better" if we could get our level of confidence even further above the action threshold, within reason. This is a valid perception that we could call "the value of knowing." It may offer true "benefit" to the patient and physician psychologically, medicolegally, or in other regards to be just "a little more sure" of things. I consider this a good reason to order more tests—sometimes. However, it should be recognized that the reasons are not quantitative and that they do not add value from a strategic viewpoint. The additional costs and confusion they may cause should be justified by the psychological benefit they provide.

It can be a tough judgment when it comes to deciding whether to order these "reassurance add-on tests." However, as I use decision analysis more and more, I have come to realize that such tests do not add as much comfort as I once believed; in fact they usually cause more trouble than they prevent. Rather, I have refined my interactions with patients so that my explanations foresee this issue and the patient becomes a supportive participant in the proper decisions to begin with. Over time, I have come to use tests of this type less and less, but they still find their place once in a while. Here is what I might say to a patient:

> "At this time, we have all the information we need to know that treatment is your best course of action. Although we cannot be sure how the situation will turn out, we can feel confident that your best decision is to proceed with treatment."

> "You asked about doing more tests to increase our confidence level. These tests would not change our mind about treatment being the best decision. Plus, they may turn up unexpected and confusing results that may muddy the waters. If it were me, I would feel comfortable taking treatment at this time without further tests."

At this time, the somewhat elusive concept of uncertainty can now be managed more readily. It can be seen from the example of the "lottery" that the right decision can be determined regardless of whether there are 51 or 99 black marbles in the basket. We can live with this wide range of uncertainty—both in lotteries and in medicine—because we have decided where the threshold lies.

You can now think about treatment in terms of just how sure you need to be about the diagnosis before the treatment becomes the "best bet." This implies knowing the diagnostic likelihood before deciding. The next chapter addresses such issues.

Chapter 5

DISEASE LIKELIHOOD AND TESTS

—⚬⚬⚬—

In the earlier chapters, we discussed how important it is to estimate the likelihood of a diagnosis: This information is necessary to decide whether to treat or not. Estimating disease likelihood before and after performing diagnostic tests is traditionally called *Bayesian analysis*. This chapter is about Bayesian thinking, but with a few interesting twists to make it easier and more natural.

There are two times when we normally make estimates of disease likelihood:

1. When we first see the patient, before doing significant diagnostic tests

2. After the results of the tests are back

MAKING A PRE-TEST ESTIMATE OF DISEASE LIKELIHOOD

It is *before* testing that one typically starts making a clinical decision. The patient presents to the physician, and one or more diagnoses are considered. Often, there is little doubt about the correct diagnosis—in decision analysis terms, the clinician has a high pre-test estimate for the likelihood of the index disease. In referring to the pre-test estimate, we are assuming that important diagnostic test results are not yet available and that we have at our disposal only the history, physical examination, and perhaps a few simple office laboratory test results.

How do we come up with pre-test estimates? In general, we rely on knowledge, experience, and judgment. We have a rough sense of the epidemiology of the disease (corrected for the risk profile of the individual patient), and then we correct for the specifics of the presentation. We consider how specific the presenting findings are for the index disease; how many different independent findings suggestive of the disease are present; and at what risk the individual patient is for the disease in question. Finally, we involuntarily rely on our past experience with the disease to develop an intuitive "feeling" for its likelihood. In the end, there is much we do not know about how physicians arrive at a diagnosis, but these are some of the things we take into consideration. Overall we do quite well.

A fine source for estimating the prevalence of disease is the evidence pertaining to diagnostic tests. Cohort studies often contain groups of patients who represent the population you would typically suspect of a disease; they also receive the gold standard test for that disease prospectively (that is, after they are assigned to the groups). As long as that population reasonably reflects your patient, the prevalence may serve as a starting point. Then again, it may be highly atypical, such as a tertiary care center's referral base; your own judgment must guide you as to how applicable the data are.

By the way, having a rough sense of the epidemiology of a disease is an area most of us need to work on; we resort to a guess in this area far more readily than we would in other areas of decision making. Next time you read about a disease, don't jump right to the treatment section—learn just how common it is in patients you are likely to see. For example, in one study of patients reporting that they believed that they had sinusitis, more than 30% actually did, as proved by radiographs and sinus aspirate cultures (5). Given specific findings, the number jumped to more than 50%. Most colleagues I questioned informally have guessed a much lower number.

The intellectual shortcuts that physicians use in this process have been called "**heuristics.**" The main reason for discussing them here is to point out that there are a few heuristics that can be problematic and thus tend to distort our estimates. By understanding and avoiding these "traps," you can make your estimates more accurate.

TRAPS TO AVOID IN PRE-TEST ESTIMATION OF DISEASE LIKELIHOOD

Trap: Because you have recently seen a case or two of an unusual disease, you overestimate the likelihood of that disease in the next patient who presents with a few of its findings, even though more common diseases are far more likely to cause the same symptoms.

> **Example**: Dr. Watson has just seen a case of Wilson's disease of the liver, an uncommon but serious and treatable cause of liver enzyme abnormalities. One week later, a 45-year-old businessman who enjoys "four or five" cocktails per day comes in for a physical and is noted to have a mild elevation of a sensitive liver enzyme. Dr. Watson thinks of Wilson's disease, even though he realizes it is a rare entity with a likelihood that he estimates is "less than 1%." Nevertheless, knowing the seriousness of the disease he decides to screen for it with an expensive serum ceruloplasmin level.
>
> **Comment**: In fact, Wilson's disease has a prevalence of only about 1 in 1,000,000 (6). Even with a mild abnormality of the blood test as the only finding, its prevalence in patients older than 30 years of age in the absence of other findings is likely to be even lower. The cost to find a single case using this strategy would run millions of dollars, and many abnormals would turn out to be false positives, creating much anxiety and additional cost.
>
> Dr. Watson should have recognized that the diagnosis was prominent in his mind because he had recently seen a case, and he should have recalled the true low prevalence of the disease; he should have reserved screening for the proper age group and in the presence of additional findings such as Kaiser-Fleischer rings and other characteristic findings. This has been called the **"availability heuristic."**

Trap: You see a constellation of common findings, which, taken together, are highly representative of a specific diagnosis. However, that diagnosis is so rare and the findings are so common that you overestimate the diagnostic likelihood.

> **Example:** Dr. Welby sees a patient (an avid gardener), apparently in good health and with no known risk factors, for a routine physical examination. As an incidental finding he notes several splinter hemorrhages under the nails of both hands, and a small ecchymosis on the sole of the right foot consistent with a Janeway lesion. In addition, a grade II/VI pulmonic ejection murmur is heard. The patient had her teeth cleaned 6 weeks earlier. Somewhat concerned about what he estimates as a "2% to 3%" chance of subacute bacterial endocarditis, Dr. Welby orders three blood cultures.
>
> **Comment:** Dr. Welby was misled by the typicality or "representativeness" of the findings; indeed they were quite representative of the classic findings of endocarditis. The problem is that they are also common findings of other conditions (e.g., trauma from gardening, functional murmur); endocarditis is a rare disease in the absence of known risk factors, and these incidental findings are far more likely to be due to other causes.
>
> Dr. Welby would have been better advised to look up the disease in the literature to refresh his memory. Although the findings jogged him to think about subacute bacterial endocarditis, the disease has an incidence of approximately 2 per 100,000, almost always is associated with fever (95%) and anorexia (98%), and usually occurs in

patients with identifiable risk factors (7). The likelihood of subacute endocarditis in this patient is therefore extremely low. This has been called the **"representative heuristic."**

Being "off" by 10% or more is often perfectly acceptable—it may not affect your final decision about testing or treating. However, being off by a factor of 100 or 1000, as in the examples just given, is clearly something to avoid and is usually the result of either failure to look up the facts or flawed reasoning. You can easily train yourself to avoid these pitfalls; indeed we owe it to our patients to do so. In the end, however, it must be acknowledged that there will always be situations where all one can do is guess.

UNCERTAINTY IN PRE-TEST ESTIMATIONS OF DISEASE LIKELIHOOD

All this may sound a bit daunting. With so much riding on our pre-test estimates, how could our ultimate decisions possibly be reliable, given the difficulties in making such estimates? Actually, if one avoids the usual pitfalls, pre-test estimates can be quite good. It is uncommon for an "error" of a few percentage points to affect one's decision, and even then there are ways of assessing a decision over a *range* of likelihoods to see if the decision holds up. An important step is to know the prevalence rates of a given disease in general.

A sound strategy is to come up with a *high* and *low* limit of pre-test likelihoods over which you can feel confident, then test your decision to see if further refinement is necessary. That is, rather than saying a disease is 20% likely, one can say it is probably *approximately* 20% likely but may be as unlikely as 10% or as likely as 30%; within that range one may feel comfortable that the "true" likelihood will be captured. If the final decision (as discussed later) changes as you move within the range, it may be necessary to do a first round of tests to narrow things down, then do further tests to refine your decision. This will often not be necessary, because the pre-test decision will remain unchanged over the entire range of likelihoods that you have defined. Testing your assumptions over a range of values is called **sensitivity analysis**.

DIAGNOSTIC TESTING

Consider a patient in whom you suspect a given diagnosis based on the history and physical examination plus your baseline knowledge of the disease.

Graphically, it may look like the diagram shown in Figure 5-1.

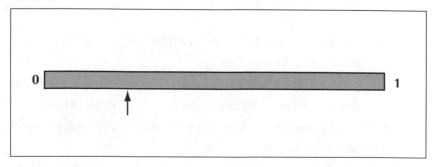

Figure 5-1. A typical diagram for demonstrating decision thresholds begins with a probability bar and an arrow representing the pre-test estimate of likelihood.

In this figure, the bar represents probability of disease in a patient or in a population, from 0 (no possibility of disease at all) on the left, to 1 (disease is certainly present) on the right. The small, upward-pointing arrow is our pre-test estimate of disease likelihood, in this example 0.2 or 20%.

You now want to refine your hypothesis—either to rule out a disease you did not suspect strongly or to rule in a disease you did suspect strongly. A positive test result will increase the pre-test estimate of disease likelihood to a predictable level (the positive predictive value), and a negative test will decrease the likelihood of disease to a predictable level (1 minus the negative predictive value, because the negative predictive value is actually the probability of *health*— *not disease*—after a negative result).

"Good" tests can dramatically improve our pre-test estimates, particularly if the estimate was in an intermediate range to begin with (the changes in disease likelihood that result from testing tend to be lower as the pre-test estimate approaches the higher or lower extremes). Because virtually all tests in actual usage are imperfect, every test leaves us with some uncertainty regardless of the result.

Figure 5-2 illustrates how the diagram in Figure 5-1 may appear after a test is completed.

Now a "spread" line has been added to the pre-test estimate arrow. At the left side, it extends down to the new probability after a negative result. To the right, it extends to the positive predictive value.

These three points correspond to the pre-test probability of disease (the arrow, approximately 25%), the post-test estimate of disease likelihood after a *negative* test result (around

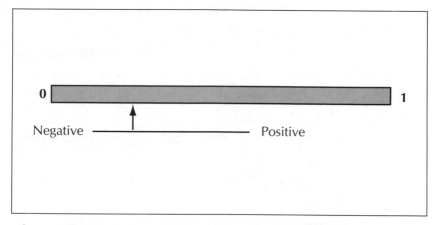

Figure 5-2. The horizontal line below the probability bar represents how much a positive or negative test result changes the pre-test estimate of disease likelihood.

15%), and the post-test estimate of disease likelihood after a *positive* result (around 60%). **This is the essence of how diagnostic tests work: They modify our pre-test estimate** by a greater or lesser amount, depending on the power of the test. Note that, in general, tests do not "make a diagnosis"—*you* do, based on the test result *in the context of how likely you believed the disease was to begin with.* This is important: think about a "positive" sedimentation rate result of 60 or so. For a patient with striking symptoms of polymyalgia rheumatica who is in the right age and risk groups it may be almost diagnostic; for a low-risk patient it may be meaningless. Other than so-called "pathognomonic" tests (if only we had more of them!), which are often invasive and expensive, few tests are diagnostic by themselves.

The next section discusses how to define and use the power of tests.

LIKELIHOOD RATIOS

Recall the definitions of sensitivity and specificity, which are the traditional parameters used to measure the power of a test. Sensitivity and specificity use the *probability* form of likelihood.

Sensitivity: the probability that a test will be positive *when the index disease is present.*

Specificity: the probability that a test will be negative *when the index disease is absent.*

Isn't it ironic that both parameters measure the power of the test "when the disease is present," or "when the disease is absent?" *If we knew whether the disease was present, we wouldn't be doing the test!* However, there is a better way of measuring the power of the test: **likelihood ratios**. From both a logical and an operational perspective, likelihood ratios have advantages over sensitivity and specificity *because they use the **odds** form of likelihood*:

> **Likelihood ratio (positive test results)**: how much more likely a diagnosis is after a positive test result compared with its likelihood before the test.
>
> **Likelihood ratio (negative test results)**: how much less likely a diagnosis is after a negative test result compared with its likelihood before the test.
>
> **Post-test odds** are simply **pre-test odds** multiplied by the **likelihood ratio** of the test:

$$\text{Post-test Odds} = \text{Pre-test Odds} \times \text{Likelihood Ratio}$$

Compare this to the formula for positive predictive value (the formula for negative predictive value is equally cumbersome):

$$\text{Positive Predictive Value} = \frac{\text{Sensitivity} \times \text{Pre-test Probability}}{(\text{Sensitivity} \times \text{Pre-test Probability}) + (1 - \text{Specificity}) \times (1 - \text{Pre-test Probability})}$$

You do not need to know this formula because the odds–likelihood ratio form is much simpler to recall and to use.

Example: Consider an exercise stress test for significant coronary disease. Its likelihood ratio (positive test result) is 2.4 and its likelihood ratio (negative test result) is 0.23. If the pre-test odds of coronary disease were 0.25, after the patient took a stress test the post-test odds of coronary disease after a positive test result would be 0.25×2.4, or 0.6, and after a negative test result would be 0.25×0.23, or 0.06. Calculate using odds and, if desired, convert your answer to probability.

The formulas for likelihood ratios are easy (use the 0-to-1 scale for sensitivity and specificity):

$$\text{Likelihood Ratio (+)} = \frac{\text{Sensitivity}}{1 - \text{Specificity}}$$

$$\text{Likelihood Ratio (–)} = \frac{1 - \text{Sensitivity}}{\text{Specificity}}$$

and

$$\text{Post-test Odds} = \text{Pre-test Odds} \times \text{Likelihood Ratio}$$

Use a positive likelihood ratio when the test is positive, and a negative likelihood ratio when the result is negative. Logically, positive likelihood ratios are always greater than 1, and negative likelihood ratios are less than 1; otherwise the test would not be rational.

TEST DISUTILITY

Although most of the tests we perform are benign for the patient (other than in terms of their costs), some are not. In particular, angiography, endoscopy, and certain biopsies entail discomfort or risk. The factor used to quantify this effect is called disutility. Usually it is of minimal impact, but if a disutility is present, its effect is to narrow the range of disease likelihood within which testing is indicated; you would be more likely simply to treat or to observe than if such a disutility were not present. We will not deal with this mathematically, but you should keep it in mind.

SUMMARY

You now have the tools to judge:

1. The likelihood of the diagnosis that would justify treatment as the best course of action (harm, improvement, and the action threshold discussed in earlier chapters).

2. The estimate of disease likelihood before testing and the estimate of disease likelihood after testing, based on

whether the test results are positive or negative (pre-test estimate of disease likelihood, likelihood ratios, and post-test estimate of disease likelihood).

It follows that you can use these skills together. The next chapter discusses how to do so in the context of making clinical decisions.

Chapter 6

CLINICAL DECISIONS: UNIFYING THE CONCEPTS

—∞∞∞—

Let us examine what we have discussed in earlier chapters in a new way (new for this book, but introduced in the medical literature [8] as early as 1980).

Consider a typical clinical scenario in which we suspect a diagnosis for which there exists a reasonable treatment. We are not certain of the diagnosis but have tests available. Before we do anything, our judgment suggests which of the "big three" courses of action (treat, observe, or test) we would be inclined to select.

One thing we desire from a test is *the power to confirm our pretest decision*. If our pre-test estimate of the disease likelihood is higher than the action threshold (such that we are inclined to treat), our hope is that the test will confirm this decision. That way, all the "ducks are in a row" and the treatment is undertaken with confidence.

We also use tests to advantage when they *have the power to change our mind*. The test results may be such that they make us lose confidence in our original hypothesis and prevent us from proceeding the way we might have before we had done the tests. In this case, the test results go against our initial inclination, so we may need a little more convincing.

If we had to choose between two tests, it is usually in our patients' interest to choose the one which would be strongest at changing our decision. Emotionally, we would rather see our suspicions confirmed than overturned, but there is more decision value in a test whose power to alter our decision is the highest. Similarly, if that same test confirmed our suspicion, our confidence would be high.

Figure 6-1 illustrates how this scenario may appear in a diagram. In this figure, the pre-test estimate is a bit below the action threshold; a positive result would take us above the action threshold.

This leads us to the following central conclusions:

• If our pre-test estimate is *below* the action threshold, we would be inclined to observe—that is, not to treat. **In order to be useful to the patient, any test we select must be powerful enough such that, given our pre-test estimate, a positive result will raise our suspicion of disease *above* the action threshold.** In other words, the test should have the power to change our preliminary decision. If even a positive result would leave the likelihood below the action threshold, the test would not be useful (we would still observe rather than treat).

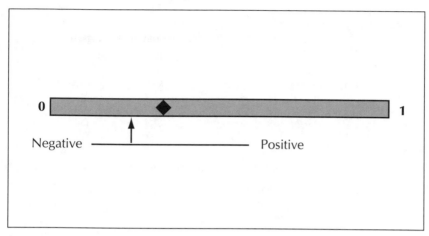

Figure 6-1. The diagram in Figures 5-1 and 5-2 (for showing the impact of tests) now includes a black diamond within the bar, representing the action threshold. We thus have the pre-test estimate of likelihood (↑), the post-test estimates of likelihood (horizontal line), and the action threshold.

• If our pre-test estimate is *above* the action threshold, we would be inclined to treat. As before, any test we select must be powerful enough such that, given our pre-test estimate, a negative result will decrease our suspicion of disease below the action threshold. If a negative result still would leave the likelihood above the action threshold, the test would not be useful (we still would treat).

A Brief Digression: A potential source of confusion when you see all of these concepts in one diagram is determining at what stage of an analysis each one is used. The concepts can be categorized as follows:

Used Before Testing	Used After Testing
Pre-test estimate of disease likelihood	Post-test estimate of disease likelihood
Likelihood ratios of tests	**Action threshold**
Action threshold	

Note that (1) most of the brainwork occurs before testing, and (2) only the action threshold has importance in both lists.

We have now addressed all of the important principles underlying a bedside decision analysis. We will next discuss how to proceed in a stepwise fashion in real-world situations.

STEPS TO FOLLOW IN A DECISION ANALYSIS

Here are the basic steps you follow to make a sound decision if you are doing it "in your head" rather than by computer (using odds to make the math easier):

1. Make a clinical estimate (before testing) of the likelihood of the disease as odds.

    Clue: Odds = Probability / (1 – Probability)

2. Estimate or calculate the action threshold for the treatment you would advise. Use your patient's subjective preferences in estimating the impact of the various outcomes. You may wish to convert your action threshold to odds, as you will see in a moment.

Clue: Harm = Probability of harm times its impact score

Clue: Improvement = Probability of improvement of disease multiplied by its impact score.

Clue: Action threshold = Harm/Improvement (as probability)

3. Select the test that best suits the scenario if more than one test is available. Seek the test that has the greatest power to change your mind; if your pre-test estimate is *above* the action threshold, choose the test with the lowest *negative* likelihood ratio (rule-out). If it is *below* the action threshold, select the test with the highest *positive* likelihood ratio (rule-in).

    These are just "the numbers." If a given test entails disutility such as great cost, risk, pain, or other negative implications, clinical judgment (the final arbiter of all things clinical) may rightfully override the mathematically "correct" decision in favor of a more humane one.

4. Calculate what the post-test estimates of likelihood would be if the test results were positive and if the test results were negative.

    Clue: Post-test Odds = Pre-test Odds × Likelihood Ratio

5. If your test would take you from below the action threshold (pre-test odds) to above the action threshold (post-test odds) or from above the action threshold to below the action threshold, go ahead and test. If it would not do so, there is no point in testing because the test results would not change your mind.

6. Based on the actual test result, if your post-test estimate of disease likelihood is above the action threshold, treat. If below, observe.

Summary of Decision Strategies

	Post-test estimate of likelihood is below action threshold	Post-test estimate of likelihood is above action threshold
Pre-test estimate of likelihood is below action threshold	Observe	Test (treat if test result is positive, observe if test result is negative)
Pre-test estimate of likelihood is above action threshold	Test (treat if test result is positive, observe if test result is negative)	Treat

---

The summary of decision strategies is included on a pocket-sized card in Appendix C on p 107.

TRAPS TO AVOID IN MAKING DECISIONS

It is not uncommon for doctors to do a test, get the results, and persist in taking a course of action that defies the results.

Trap: Ignoring a negative test result.

Example: Dr. Watson sees a patient who "seems" to have strep throat. He decides to do a strep screen, the results of which turn out to be negative, and yet he treats with penicillin anyhow.

Comment: Although there may have been nothing wrong with the decision to treat, it causes one to wonder why Dr. Watson bothered doing the test. If the pre-test estimate was so high that even a negative result would leave enough suspicion of strep to warrant treatment, the test was not worth doing. Community and household contact welfare aside, this is an illogical approach.

Trap: Ignoring a positive test result.

Example: Dr. Welby sees a 59-year-old man who has one of three fecal occult blood cards turn up positive in a screening setting. Dr. Welby decides that this may well be owing to benign factors and advises the patient to "repeat the test in a few months."

Comment: Dr. Welby recognized that the test was imperfect, but according to the evidence (9), its flaw lies in its mediocre negative likelihood ratio (approximately 0.24 to 0.64, depending on the type of testing done) and not in its positive likelihood ratio (approximately 6 to 18). Whether fecal occult blood testing is a suitable screening test is controversial, but once it has been carried out and the results are *positive*, the post-test estimate of likelihood of colon cancer or adenomatous polyp (assuming conservatively a prevalence of 7% and a positive likelihood ratio of 6) is about 30%, high enough to warrant colonoscopy. Why perform the test if a positive result is going to be ignored; why delay intervention?

Assess a test as worthwhile or not worthwhile using the principles discussed. If you decide it is worth doing, stick to your guns when the results are in.

I hope that a keener understanding of decision making will lead to a reduction in such innumerate decisions.

KEEPING DECISION ANALYSIS PRACTICAL

Because it is unrealistic to expect any busy practitioner to perform even a simple decision analysis dozens of times a day, here are some strategies you may consider:

- Don't bother with formal analysis for every patient for noncritical clinical treatments. Many decisions are self-evident to a thoughtful doctor (notwithstanding the cautionary examples we have just discussed). For significant treatment decisions, however, take five minutes to do the estimates and calculations.

- For treatments that are fairly trivial (are they ever trivial to the patient?) but are common in your practice, calculate an action threshold using utilities that you believe are sensible and reflective of your typical patient. Use these for formulating your *strategies* toward these problems. Although the utilities may not be individualized, you can verify them with the patient when needed, and at least you will have a sensible baseline from which to start. Similarly, collect the likelihood ratios of commonly performed tests for these same conditions for easy reference (see Appendix E on pp 110 and 111 for templates to help you organize this information).

- For decisions in which major issues are at stake, consider performing a formal analysis or obtaining consultation from someone capable of doing one. After all, your patient has a great deal riding on it.

USE A COMPUTER PROGRAM

A computer program can streamline the process; it allows you to simply select the disease, test, and treatment and provides instant analyses of the type described here along with several others.

In addition, the test and treatment data (such as likelihood), which are not always readily available at the bedside or in the examination room, can be stored within the program database itself. The program can also display the resulting analyses graphically so that you can gain an intuitive grasp of the process each time you vary any parameter. Furthermore, by allowing instant recalculation, users can test their conclusions over any range of estimates, thus doing a "sensitivity analysis" in seconds. See Appendix D on p 109 for details about such a program.

ROLL YOUR OWN COMPUTER PROGRAM

You do not need a special program to do most of this work; a simple spreadsheet will suffice, even on a hand-held device. Figure 6-2 is an example of a spreadsheet you can use.

Spreadsheet Decision Analysis Engine

1		Probability	Odds
2	**Pre-test estimate**	?	= B2/(1 − B2)
3			
4	**Test sensitivity**	?	= B4/(1 − B4)
5	**Test specificity**	?	= B5/(1 − B5)
6			
7	**Harm probability**	?	= B7/(1 − B7)
8	**Harm impact**	?	
9			
10	**Improvement probability**	?	= B10/(1 − B10)
11	**Improvement impact**	?	
12		Odds	Probability
13	**Likelihood ratio (positive)**	= B4/(1 − B5)	= B13/(1 + B13)
14	**Likelihood ratio (negative)**	= (1 − B4)/B5	= B14/(1 + B14)
15	**Post-test estimate of likelihood (test result positive)**	= C2 × B13	= C15/(1 + C15)
16	**Post-test estimate of likelihood (test result negative)**	= C2 × B14	= B16/(1 + B16)
17	**Action threshold**		= (B7 × B8)/(B10 × B11)

Figure 6-2. Enter these formulas in your favorite spreadsheet. You may have to alter the syntax to conform to the program you use. The cells with "?" are entered by the user, and the remainder are calculated by the program. Using such a program in a hand-held device makes bedside decision-making fast and easy. "Power users" may even be able to add a conditional interpretation row based on the Summary of Decision Strategies table on p 70.

Note: Row numbers are provided for clarity and may or may not appear in your software; column 1 is the description column. The odds and probabilities columns reverse order at row 12 because the order of calculation requires this (probabilities are calculated after the odds for these rows).

Chapter 7

EXAMPLES OF CLINICAL DECISION MAKING

———∞∞∞———

The following examples are provided to help you incorporate the concepts in the earlier chapters in a clinically meaningful way. The data provided are illustrative and are not intended to be authoritative.

EXAMPLE 1: STREP THROAT

Mrs. White presents with a sore throat for 36 hours. On physical examination she has a temperature of 38.5 °C and bilateral tonsillar exudates but no adenopathy or other findings. Her history is entirely unremarkable otherwise. You must decide whether to

1. Provide symptomatic treatment only or no treatment

2. Perform a test for strep and act according to the results

3. Provide treatment with penicillin, without testing.

Step 1: Pre-test estimate. Based on the findings described above, you know that your pre-test estimate for the likelihood of strep throat is in the 20% range. If no exudate or fever were present, it would be less than 10%; if tender anterior adenopathy were present in addition to the other two findings, it would be more than 40% (10).

Step 2: Estimating the action threshold. Oral penicillin is a benign drug. Estimate its **harm** as follows: approximately 4% of patients develop either an uncomfortable rash or diarrhea; anaphylaxis is so rare as to not be a factor in the decision (<1:200,000); other serious allergic reactions occur in fewer than 1% of patients. The "impact" of diarrhea or rash for 2 to 3 days for this patient (Mrs. White) is estimated to be quite low, perhaps 0.1 on a 0-to-1 scale. Thus,

$$\text{Harm frequency} = 5\%$$
$$\text{Harm impact} = 0.1$$

The **improvements** of penicillin relate to a reduction in sore throat of about 2 days in virtually all patients with strep throat and prevention of peritonsillar abscesses in approximately 5%; there is some reduction in risk for rheumatic fever and glomerulonephritis, but the incidence of both of these in adults is very low.

Let's estimate the **impact** for preventing 2 days of sore throat. Keeping in mind that we rated several days of diarrhea or rash at a 0.1 impact, we should now *compare* the impact of sore throat (prevented) to that of rash or diarrhea. We can add a little extra impact for the occasional abscess we might prevent, but this would be small. Because harm impact (e.g., rash, diarrhea) was 0.1, we may estimate *improvement* impact to be fairly similar at 0.1. That is, a day with a bad sore throat is about the same as (i.e., as bad as) a day with rash or diarrhea, in the patient's opinion. The actual numbers we choose are not crucial. What is crucial is to keep the *ratio* between the impacts consistent with the patient's feelings. You might judge it differently, and that is just the point: It should reflect the *patient's* values.

> **Example:** Suppose that your patient is a swimsuit model. Although he or she could still work passably well with a sore throat or even with diarrhea (albeit with some inconvenience), a visible rash would put the patient out of commission for a while. The patient thus rates the impact of a rash much higher than he or she would rate the impact of a sore throat. In that case, the "harm" impact would have to be increased a bit, thus raising the action threshold. This admittedly contrived example illustrates how individual patient *utilities* affect your estimate of harm and improvement.

Thus,

$$\text{Improvement frequency} = 1$$
$$\text{Improvement impact} = 0.1$$

The **action threshold** for penicillin–strep throat (Harm/Improvement) is thus:

$$(0.1 \times 0.05)/(0.1 \times 1)$$

This corresponds to a probability of .05 or 5%. That is, if you were 5% confident of a strep throat, you would treat knowing that this would be the best decision.

Step 3: Assessing Testing. Because your pre-test estimate (20%, or odds of 0.25) is above the action threshold (5%, or odds of 1:19), you may be inclined simply to treat. However, we need to know if a test could change your mind. We know that throat cultures have a sensitivity of approximately 90% (relative to acute antibody titer increases as the gold standard). Specificity is about 85% (many patients harbor GABH strep as normal flora) (8). This translates to a positive likelihood ratio of [0.9/(1–0.85)], or 6, and a negative likelihood ratio of [(1–0.9)/0.85], or 0.12. Here is what we have so far, using formulas discussed elsewhere:

	Probability	Odds
Pre-test estimate of likelihood	20%	0.25
Likelihood ratios (positive and negative)		6, 0.12
Action threshold	5%	0.052
Post-test estimate of likelihood (positive test result)	67%	1.5
Post-test estimate of likelihood (negative test result)	3%	0.03

Step 4: Interpreting the test results. Testing would change your pre-test estimate of strep throat from 20% to 3% if the result were negative. Because this clearly crosses the action threshold of 5%, the test has value: It could change your mind about whether or not to treat.

Step 5: Confirming the pre-test estimate. Maybe your pre-test estimate is not quite right. Maybe your harm or improvement estimates are not as good as you would like them to be. This is not a problem—simply repeat the process using different numbers (this is where the spreadsheet provided earlier comes in handy). If your decision holds up, your confidence in your decision will increase. If not, it may be too close a call to rely on one test; in this case, you should consider further testing or rethinking your assumptions.

EXAMPLE 2: CAROTID BRUIT

Here is a more complex case. It illustrates how to interpret "best" evidence when "perfect" evidence does not exist.

A 60-year-old man (without atherosclerotic risk factors) was noted to have an asymptomatic carotid bruit on routine examination. You consider the possible actions to take: ignoring it, performing ultrasonography, or referring directly for angiography with possible endarterectomy. You perform a computer literature review (it took me 20 minutes to do this in real time). The data are highly controversial and, by the way, are likely to change in the near future, but let's dive in just to reinforce the process:

Step 1: Making the pre-test estimate. The disease we are discussing is 60% or greater occlusion—that is, the degree of internal carotid stenosis for which endarterectomy usually benefits patients. Let us be careful to assess the risk of this in patients *with asymptomatic bruits*, not in those with previous transient ischemic attack, stroke, and so on, as discussed in much of the literature.

Lewis and colleagues (11) report a prevalence range of about 2% to 13% for stenosis of 50% or more, depending on risk profile. This is not precisely what we need (60% stenosis, no risks, male), but many of the patients in this study had multiple risk factors, so it is reasonable to accept 5% as a sensible "best estimate" for the pre-test likelihood in this lower-risk patient. Bruits are found in approximately 5% of 65-year-old men (12), but a bruit, although a relative risk for strokes in general, probably increases the likelihood of high-grade stenosis by only a small amount (e.g., from 52% to 63% in *symptomatic* patients). Therefore, 5% to 6% pre-test probability for high-grade stenosis in this patient seems to hold up, bruit and all. We won't quibble over a percent or two.

Step 2: Estimating the action threshold. Fortunately, a thoughtful decision analysis was found that summarized many of the numbers we need (13). Because both endarterectomy and angiography carry risk, let's combine the risk of the two interventions: 0.007 for angiography (death or serious stroke) and 0.018 for endarterectomy (myocardial infarction, death, major stroke), for a total of 0.025 or 2.5% *immediate* disaster for the **harm frequency**. Our patient needs to assess the collective impact of this group of outcomes (myocardial infarction, death, and serious stroke) on a 0-to-1 scale. Let's use a **harm impact** that reflects their gravity—say, 0.9.

To estimate improvement, if the disease is more than 60% occlusion and if the patient does not undergo surgery (that is, the disease is not treated), the annual death rate per year will be 3.5% (compared with 3% with surgery) and the rate of nonfatal major stroke will be 1.5% (compared with 0.06% with surgery). Extended over 5 years, this gives a cumulative risk of death of 17.5% for patients who do not receive treatment compared with 15% for those who do receive treatment, and a risk of serious stroke of 7.5% for patients who do not receive treatment compared with 0.3% for those who do receive treatment. So, treatment yields a 2.5% 5-year improvement in mortality and a 7.2% improvement in the rate of serious strokes, for a total of 9.7% major **improvement frequency** (most of which is stroke prevention). Again, a patient who has benefited from the treatment would estimate improvement to be quite high but spread over 5 years. Because we rated harm to be 0.9 when there were similar *immediate* outcomes, we would have to give a somewhat lower impact score to these when they are spread over 5 years—say, a 0.6 (there are formal ways of comparing immediate risk to risk spread over time, but let's satisfy ourselves with subjective estimates for now).

We can summarize as follows:

$$\text{Harm} = 0.025 \times 0.9 \ = 0.0225$$
$$\text{Improvement} = 0.097 \times 0.6 \ = 0.0582$$
$$\text{Action Threshold} = 0.0225 / 0.0492 = 0.39$$

This means that if you were more than 39% confident in the diagnosis of internal carotid stenosis (60% occlusion), treatment would be your best bet.

Step 3: Assessing testing. Ultrasonography for 70% stenosis of the left internal carotid has a sensitivity of 88% and a specificity of 90% (14). The likelihood ratio (positive test result) thus equals $0.88/(1–0.9)$, or 8.8.

Thus, here is what we have so far:

	Probability	Odds
Pre-test likelihood	5%	1:19
Likelihood ratios (positive and negative)		8.8, 0.13
Action threshold	39%	0.64
Post-test likelihood (positive test result)	44%	0.67

Step 4: Interpreting the test results. Because a positive test result would increase the likelihood of disease from 5% to 44%, it would indeed take it across the action threshold (39%). Thus, if the results of ultrasonography were positive, the patient would be better off undergoing angiography with possible endarterectomy.

Conclusion: Test, then treat only if the result is positive.

COMMENTS

This is a pretty close call: If our post-test likelihood were just a bit lower, it would change the decision. I hope you are uncomfortable with this—it is too close to rely on, being based on some highly subjective assumptions we made about utilities and pre-test estimates. In such cases, you should rework the analysis using *ranges* for these parameters that fall within reasonable limits. For example, if you are not sure about the 5% pre-test estimate, try 13% instead (the upper limit in the literature search).

If you continue to waver in your interpretation, call it a draw and recognize that you have reached the limits of this technique. Many would opt not to do anything if the relative advantages are that marginal. On the other hand, if your decision solidifies over most of the ranges you use, you can feel comfortable that your decision is sound.

For completeness, a study by Hobson (15) measured actual *outcomes* in asymptomatic men who were screened and *shown to have high-grade stenosis* (a much higher risk group than that of the patient described in the above example). Even in *that* population, intervention failed to show overall improvement for patients who underwent the surgery. This is a more powerful argument against intervention than our decision analysis.

Limitations of our analysis include that we had to "lump together" the combined outcomes of death and serious stroke into a single impact score. This may not be wise for a patient who would judge death to have *much* more impact than a serious stroke. Fortunately the same process occurred on both the harm and improvement side, so some "offsetting" effect is involved. Also, note that we judged the impact of *immediate* harm (perioperative) as more important than *delayed* improvement (occurring over a period of 5 years). This is not uncommon and should always be considered.

As an exercise, consider that very high-risk groups (e.g., older males with hypertension who smoke heavily and have a bruit) may have high-grade stenosis 50% of the time (pre-test estimate of likelihood). Repeat the process above and see what you come up with. *Hint*: you might still cross the action threshold, but in reverse.

CONCLUSION

The elegance of decision analysis sometimes gets lost in the details. However, if you realize that it gives you a way of dealing with uncertainty while assuring that your reasoning is logically and quantitatively consistent, you can appreciate the powerful effect it can and should have on your clinical practice.

To be sure, much room for error remains even when you apply this approach; data can be invalid, presumptions and estimates can be wrong, human error will always rear its head. But that error potential exists with or without a bedside decision analysis; if you compound it by superimposing flawed reasoning, the results can only be worse. It is best to use decision analysis whenever possible and worry about the evidence, not the process.

The reader is encouraged to incorporate the concepts of decision analysis into his or her practice. Even if you rely on estimates and do not process every step in a formal way, it will clarify your thinking. Optimally, the conscientious application of decision analysis to every nontrivial clinical decision should be carried out whenever a patient's welfare might be affected.

Chapter 8

DECISION TREES 101

WHERE DO DECISION TREES BELONG?

It was stated earlier that you will usually defer the use of decision trees to those who are experienced with the tool, and that it takes considerable practice to use trees effectively. For most decisions you are likely to face in clinical practice, the use of decision trees is either unnecessary or impractical. In that case, you may be asking, why give decision trees their own chapter?

- Decision trees appear in the literature with some regularity (in cost-effectiveness analyses as well as in clinical papers). Without a basic understanding of their "anatomy and physiology," it is not practical to critically appraise these articles.

- The act of drawing a decision tree sometimes yields important insights into the problem at hand. It forces you to be explicit about the scenario, and often makes clear certain alternative strategies that would not otherwise occur to you.

- Practice guidelines and clinical pathways often look like decision trees. However, they usually are not, and it is critical to recognize the difference. True decision trees are thoughtful, quantitative analyses, whereas the former are often simply diagrams with a branching structure. You should never confuse the two, lest you interpret a guideline as an analysis or vice versa.

- Decision trees may well prove useful to you in the development of guidelines for your own organization. Knowing how to create and understand them will place you at a great advantage.

Having said this, I must acknowledge that even without understanding the concepts in this chapter, one could utilize the principles of this book without compromise. The following material is presented for those readers who would like a brief introduction to the decision trees for the reasons listed above. The references contain excellent resources for further information (8,16).

WHAT IS A DECISION TREE?

Decision trees are the most comprehensive and explicit way of organizing and "modeling" complex medical scenarios. Developed as a tool for analyzing the impact of complicated business decisions, the technique found wide acceptance in

medical circles when it was recognized that many of its principles were applicable: estimates of probability, uncertainty, and
risk assessment.

A decision tree is a diagram that represents all the important
and plausible possibilities of a clinical scenario. Into this diagram, you insert quantitative evidence: the likelihoods of certain possibilities; the utilities of various final outcomes for your
patient, and so forth. When completed, a decision tree can be a
clever means of determining which set of "forks in the road"
will lead to the highest likelihood of a "best" outcome.

> **Example:** Suppose you are on a limited budget and go to
> a new restaurant. You can choose to order either a blue
> plate special or a red plate special. The red plate special
> is consistently good (but not great). The blue plate spe-
> cial is sometimes great, but at other times is awful. You
> need to decide which special to order. Let's do it with a
> tree (Fig. 8-1):

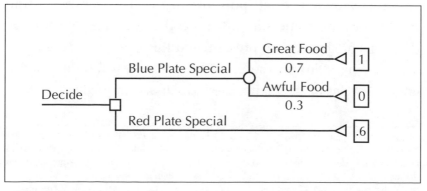

Figure 8-1. The beginnings of a decision tree. The flow goes from left to
right, top to bottom.

Here are some conventions: a square at the intersection of various branches represents a **decision node**. That is, the branch that is selected next is under your control. In the above fragment, you would decide which of the two strategies to follow: blue or red plate special.

If you chose the blue plate special, you would come to another node: great food or awful food. At this point, you lose control: the food you get is strictly a function of which chef is working, what the dish is, and so on. This node is depicted as a circle and is called a **chance node**. It shows the possible outcomes with the likelihood of each, but this is up to the whims of nature. You have no choice in the matter.

Although you cannot control the outcomes of chance nodes, you may well know something about them. In the example, numerous randomized, blinded restaurant reviewers prospectively determined that great food was served 70% of the time and awful food 30% of the time. Therefore, you know the likelihood of each outcome even when you do not have the choice.

The last type of node to understand* is the **terminal node**, which is shown as a left-pointing arrow. This represents the final logical outcome state at the end of the tree. No further decisions or chances are present, and this is where you end up after having followed the preceding branches. Terminal nodes are equivalent to the "outcomes" discussed in earlier chapters.

---

*Actually, there is another type of node: the Markov node. Although the details of this node are beyond the scope of this discussion, Markov nodes account for situations in which patients can experience one state and make a transition to a different state over time. For example, if you decide to observe patients with coronary disease rather than treat them, they may subsequently die, have a heart attack, experience worsening symptoms, or remain stable. Over time, a patient may experience several such states: stable → worse pain → death. The likelihood of such progressions is often predictable, and their utilities can be estimated. A Markov analysis estimates the aggregate utility of such complex situations within a decision tree.

As such, they can be assigned "utilities," which are in principle no different from the utilities discussed earlier. Thus, they are given a score from 0 to 1 based on personal opinion and values (as mentioned before, utility schemes such as cost and life expectancy can be used instead). In Figure 8-1, the utilities for the best and worst meal are assigned a 1 and 0, respectively. The intermediate meal is assigned (arbitrarily) a 0.6. This means I judged it to be about 60% as good as a great meal.

Look again at the figure and understand what each of its branches and numbers means. The observant reader may recognize that virtually all of these components have analogs in the threshold model discussed in previous chapters.

HOW TO CALCULATE A DECISION TREE

Now that the decision tree's anatomy has been explained, let us examine how to get the "numbers" out of it. This process, for reasons that will become clear shortly, is called "rolling back" or "folding back" the tree. The steps are as follows:

1. Starting at the topmost terminal node at the right of the tree (great food), multiply the utility by the probability of the corresponding branch. Above, this is 1×0.7, or simply 0.7. Repeat this for the other branch, which emanates from the same chance node—in this case, awful food: 0×0.3, or just 0.

2. Add the two products described above: $0.7 + 0 = 0.7$. This number is now the new utility for the "blue plate special" branch. If there were other nodes interspersed before we got to the originating branch, we would simply repeat the process of multiplying utilities and probabilities, adding

them for each chance node and proceeding leftward until we got to the original decision branch.

3. Repeat the process for all terminal nodes along with its proximal branches, if any. The red plate special branch has no chance nodes; the likelihood for a good meal is 1. Its product is thus 1×0.6, or 0.6.

You can see that each of the original branches now has a "score" that is its expected utility. This score incorporates both the utility and the probability of the various branches for that decision branch. Because the blue plate special was assigned a 0.7 and the red plate special was assigned a 0.6, the blue plate special is the winner. You will see another example of rolling back below.

WHAT DOES THE "BEST STRATEGY" ACTUALLY MEAN?

We mentioned that the blue-plate special was the "winner" in the above decision tree. This means exactly the same thing as the best decision discussed in previous chapters: It is the decision that is most likely to yield the optimal combination of probabilities and utilities for the patient. The limitations that apply to our threshold decision model are no different here—some patients choosing this strategy will do poorly, and some choosing a "lesser" strategy will do well. In the end, the preferred decision in a tree model is simply the best bet. The outcomes are not assured, but it would be unwise not to make the best bet initially.

Perhaps you can see the similarities between a decision tree and the threshold model. In fact, they are mathematically equivalent.

It is in complex scenarios that decision trees are more suitable.

A MORE COMPLEX SCENARIO

Figure 8-2 is a tree of the variety discussed in Sonnenberg's excellent article (16). It is a rather generic structure to which you can apply many clinical scenarios, and I have changed the utilities to be consistent with the units to which we are accustomed (0 to 1):

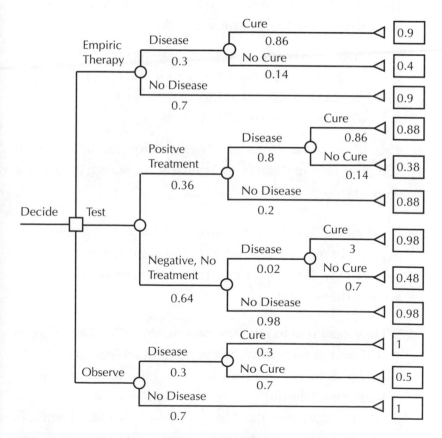

Figure 8-2. A realistic, generic medical decision tree.

Take a moment to ponder the logic of this tree. We can use it to demonstrate several points:

1. **How to roll back a more complex tree.** We can do the top terminal node as an example:

    Utility of 0.9 × Cure Probability of 0.86 = 0.77
    Utility of 0.4 × No Cure Probability of 0.14 = 0.06
    Add these two: 0.77 + 0.06 = 0.83

    These are the two branches for the Cure—No Cure chance node. That node thus assumes a utility of 0.83.

    Utility of 0.83 (from above) × Disease Probability of 0.3 = 0.25
    Utility of 0.9 (the No Disease terminal node)
      × No Disease Probability of 0.7 = 0.63
    Add these two: 0.63 × 0.25 = 0.88

    This is the final common denominator for the original "Empiric Therapy" decision branch. That branch thus gets a score of 0.88.

    An exercise: The correct answers for the remaining two decision branches (test and observe) are 0.919 and 0.895 respectively. See if you can roll back each of these to achieve those results.

2. **How easy it is to get sidetracked.** If you are like me, you will find several troubling aspects in its logic. For example, it does not account for side effects; the treatment branches "should" have "no side effects" and "side effects" branches; the "Test; Negative, No treatment; No disease" sequence has the same utility score as "Test;

Negative, No treatment; Disease–Cure" (shouldn't the presence of disease have some negative impact even if it is self-limited?); and so forth. And this is only a generic tree—add "real" disease and treatments and you can imagine how readily one can get inundated with details.

Here we see both the strength and the weakness of decision trees in "point–counterpoint":

Point: Because even moderately complex scenarios have so many possible outcomes and choices, it is nearly impossible to avoid getting profoundly lost in the medical subtleties of a tree. Try to teach decision trees to a group of physicians using real examples and you will almost certainly spend more time discussing the vagaries of the specific disease and treatment than you will the concepts of decision trees themselves.

Counterpoint: This complexity and innuendo are exactly what we face in the real world. By using a tree, these are made explicit and can be addressed directly rather than by "intuition." Besides, many subtleties that physicians bring up are of such rarity or minimal consequence that they do not affect the final analysis.

Point: So much depends on utilities, probabilities, and other numbers that it is difficult to accept a "best strategy" solution as valid. Any small change in one crucial number may change the whole recommendation. Given the complexity of the tree, the likelihood of such an occurrence cannot be dismissed.

Counterpoint: Although the point is true, with decision trees you can do virtually any "what if" revisions. Take one or more points where you doubt the number, vary it within a plausible range, and see if the conclusion holds up. At least with a decision tree you can test your conclusions in many ways; with clinical "judgment" alone, you do not have that luxury. Besides, judgment alone is often incapable of dealing with the complexity of many clinical scenarios.

Point: The process is simply too complex for routine use.

Counterpoint: True, but with computer solutions and the frequent appearance of such analyses, it behooves the thoughtful practitioner at least to understand the mechanics, strengths, and weakness of the process. Done properly, a decision tree can be a powerful tool for patients, often providing the best possible resource when randomized control trials are lacking or are not feasible.

Many other such arguments can be made, but here is a perspective on decision trees that I find to be the most helpful to practitioners:

1. Although they are too cumbersome for routine use in practice, decision trees provide a powerful and unique means of examining complex clinical scenarios. By understanding the basics, you can follow the literature when a decision tree is presented, thus making a critical appraisal of the article much more meaningful.

2. For use in caring for an individual patient, you may find that constructing a simple decision tree clarifies otherwise difficult-to-follow situations. You may sometimes incorporate the best "numbers" or evidence you can find to help you make decisions.

3. Understanding decision trees will prove invaluable as

you assess clinical guidelines in the future; you can quickly either "debunk" a pseudo-decision tree or analyze a "real" one for all it is worth.

Improperly used, decisions trees do indeed carry the risk of imbuing invalid decisions with a sort of undeserved quantitative credibility. It is only through understanding their strengths and limits that you can view them critically and clearly.

AN INTERESTING EDUCATIONAL BENEFIT

I have observed a fascinating dynamic when using decision trees in controversial clinical scenarios: When physicians disagree over the best approach to a clinical scenario, they often argue nonproductively, "This is how I have done it," or "I've had good success by doing it this way," or "No way would I take a chance on that," and so forth. By using a sound decision tree as the basis for resolving differences, however, physicians more often end up by disputing the likelihood of outcomes, the relevance of specific utilities, and other more meaningful and specific issues. It seems far more revealing, educational, and helpful to the patient to focus the arguments on what really matters: evidence and expected outcomes of alternative strategies.

CONCLUSION

I would like to immunize you against the possibility that this final chapter will leave you wondering if decision making is too confusing or cumbersome. Recalling the essential simplicity of preceding chapters, you know that you can be a good decision-maker *without* decision trees in most scenarios. Trees are useful, but they should not be allowed to confuse rather than clarify, nor should they be viewed as having any supernatural powers. As an intelligent and informed consumer, you now have the ability to judge for yourself.

EPILOGUE

—✆—

M edical decision making is a process followed by every physician for every patient. You can do it haphazardly or you can do it rationally. You can rely on experience, intuition, and subjective judgment alone, or you can enhance those important attributes with consistent, rational, and powerful tools for identifying and clarifying the decisions most likely to lead to the desired results.

Probably like you, I have had too much clinical experience to believe that decision analysis is sufficient for optimal medical care. So many intangibles weave their way throughout the patient–physician experience (thankfully!)—friendship, interpersonal skills, judgment, reassurance, hunches, experience, and other uniquely human elements too numerous and subtle to list. Yet, having used decision analysis for some time, I can no longer practice without it. Because the hailstorm of information, social and economic influences (sometimes conflicting), and patient advocacy shows no signs of abating, decision analysis has become for me a reliable anchor in the sea of uncertainty. I am pleased that you have taken the time to give it a fair assessment.

APPENDICES

APPENDIX A

GLOSSARY

Usage note: Although probabilities are percentages from 0% to 100%, most of the literature of decision analysis uses a scale of 0 to 1 instead, with 1 corresponding to 100%, 0.25 corresponding to 25%, and so on. For consistency, we shall also use the 0-to-1 scale in the following discussion.

Excellent resources exist for learning about basic medical biostatistics and epidemiology (4). Here are a selected group of definitions you may run across in the medical literature.

Action threshold—The likelihood of disease above which the given treatment is more likely to improve the condition of patients with disease than it is to harm healthy patients. It is the disease likelihood above which treatment would be the best decision, all other things being equal.

It is imperative to realize, as noted in the next section, that the action threshold for a treatment depends not only on the factual probabilities for risks and benefits of the treatment, but also on the patient's subjective preferences and fears for these various outcomes. Thus, there is no "right" or "wrong" number for the action threshold—each patient may have his or her own number.

Disutility—A negative value between 1 and 0 reflecting the harm or risk of performing the test; generally reserved for the most extreme cases.

False negative rate—The probability that a negative result will be incorrect—that is, that a patient with a negative test result may actually have the index disease. It equals 1 minus the Sensitivity.

False positive rate—The probability that a positive result will be incorrect—that is, that a patient with a positive test result actually does not have the index disease. It equals 1 minus the Specificity.

Likelihood ratio (negative test result)—The ratio of the false-negative rate to the true-negative rate; given a negative test result, it tells you how much less likely the patient is to have the disease than was estimated before the test. It assumes you are using the odds form of pre-test estimation of disease likelihood.

$$\text{Likelihood Ratio (Negative Test Result)} = \frac{1 - \text{Sensitivity}}{\text{Specificity}}$$

Likelihood ratio (positive test result)—The ratio of the true-positive rate to the false-positive rate; given a positive test result, it tells you how much more likely a patient is to have the disease than was estimated before the test. It assumes you are using the odds form of pre-test estimation of disease likelihood.

$$\text{Likelihood Ratio (Positive Test Result)} = \frac{\text{Sensitivity}}{1 - \text{Specificity}}$$

Odds—The likelihood of a condition expressed as a ratio of the affected population to the unaffected population. It is an alternate way of expressing probability.

$$\text{Probability} = \frac{\text{Odds}}{1 + \text{Odds}}$$

$$\text{Odds} = \frac{\text{Probability}}{1 - \text{Probability}}$$

Predictive value (negative test result)—The likelihood that a disease is absent given that a diagnostic test result is negative. The pre-test estimate of disease likelihood must be known in order to calculate this, along with the false-positive and false-negative rates of the test. Mnemonic: HIN = likelihood of "Healthy If Negative." This is the older way of looking at likelihood ratios and post-test estimation of disease likelihood, and is entirely dependent on knowing the prevalence rates under which it was derived.

> **Note:** In actual usage, it is usually more intuitive to consider the likelihood of disease (as opposed to that of health) given a negative result. This corresponds to 1 minus the negative predictive value.

Predictive value (positive test result)—The likelihood that a disease is present given that a diagnostic test is positive. The pre-test estimation of disease likelihood must be known in order to calculate this, along with the false-positive and false-negative rates of the test.

Pre-test estimate of disease likelihood—The odds or probability of a disease before the performance of a particular test. It generally is understood to encompass the results of history, physical examination, risk factor assessment, and sometimes minor testing.

Probability—The likelihood of a condition expressed as a percentage of the total population under consideration. It is thus a comparison of the affected population to the total population (affected + unaffected). See **Odds**, above.

Scenario—The circumstances of a clinical decision including all three cardinal factors: the disease, the test, and the treatment under consideration.

Sensitivity—The probability that a test will be positive in patients who, according to some other "gold standard," are known to have the disease in question. Mnemonic: PID = "Positive In Disease." This is synonymous with the term "True Positive Rate." SNOut = **S**ensitive tests if **N**egative rule a disease **Out**.

Specificity—The probability that a test will be negative in patients who, according to some other "gold standard," are known not to have the disease in question. It is also called the True Negative Rate. Mnemonic: NIH = "**N**egative **I**n **H**ealth." SPIn = **S**pecific tests if **P**ositive rule a disease **In**.

Testing Range—Not covered in the book explicitly, the testing range is the range of pre-test estimates of likelihood over which the best decision is to test; below this range, you would observe only, and above it, you would treat only. Using odds, it runs from: Action threshold/Likelihood ratio (positive test result) at the low end up to Action threshold/Likelihood ratio (negative test result) at the upper end.

APPENDIX B

TREATMENT EFFECTS: ADDITIONAL CONCEPTS

These terms were not discussed in the body of the manual but are often used to describe the effects of treatment. They are included here for your convenience.

Absolute risk reduction (ARR)

If a treatment reduces the probability of a particular bad disease outcome, it is said to reduce the risk for that outcome. The actual number of percentage points by which the risk is reduced is the absolute risk reduction. If warfarin reduces the risk of stroke in atrial fibrillation from 8% to 3%, the absolute risk reduction is 8% − 3%, or 5%.

Relative risk reduction (RRR)

If you express the risk reduction discussed in the definition of ARR as a fraction or proportion of the baseline risk rather than as absolute percentage points, this is called the relative risk reduction. In the example given under ARR, the 5% risk reduction would be divided by the baseline risk reduction, to give 5%/8%, or 62.5%.

It is common for various pharmaceutical and other proponents of a treatment to use relative risk reduction to make their claims "feel" larger. Never use RRR alone to assess the importance of an effect; always use RRR in conjunction with ARR.

Number needed to treat (NNT)

If you divide 100 by the ARR, you get "number needed to

treat." This represents how many patients you would need to treat in order to achieve the described improvement in a single patient. It is a useful way of looking at the ARR when you are determining the value of a treatment.

Number needed to harm (NNH)

This is the same concept as NNT but is applied to a side effect of a treatment. If the side effect occurs in 5% of patients, your NNH is 100/5, or 20. This means you would cause the side effect in 1 out of every 20 patients you treat.

APPENDIX C

POCKET GUIDE TO BEDSIDE DECISION MAKING

The Pocket Guide shown below may be copied as a reference. It is designed to fit on a standard index card.

POCKET GUIDE TO BEDSIDE DECISION MAKING

Pre-test Estimate: Use prevalence; avoid overestimating due to recent case, representativeness, and so on. Use 0 to 1 scale, convert to Odds:

$$\text{Odds} = \text{Probability}/(1 - \text{Probability})$$
$$\text{Probability} = \text{Odds}/(1 + \text{Odds})$$

Action threshold: Disease likelihood above which treatment is the "best bet."

$$\text{AT\_Probability} = \frac{\text{Harm Frequency} \times \text{Harm Impact}}{\text{Improvement Frequency} \times \text{Improvement Impact}}$$

Testing:

$\text{LR}(+) = \text{Sensitivity}/(1 - \text{Specificity})$ — *Use if test result is positive*
$\text{LR}(-) = (1 - \text{Sensitivity})/\text{Specificity}$ — *Use if test result is negative*
$\text{Post-test Odds} = \text{Pre-test Odds} \times \text{LR}$ — *Convert to probability*

Decide: Based on pre-test likelihood, post-test probability, action threshold

	If post-test estimate of likelihood < AT	If post-test estimate of likelihood > AT
If pre-test likelihood < AT	Observe	Test (treat if +, observe if –)
If pre-test likelihood > AT	Test (treat if +, observe if –)	Treat

APPENDIX D

A COMPUTER PROGRAM FOR DECISION ANALYSIS

The author has written a computer program to perform the steps outlined in this book. It also serves as a database for evidence and on-line resources. The program is called BASIS™.

The current version is for the Windows 95 or Windows 98 environments only (see the web site for other versions under development). Because the details of distribution were not available at the time of this printing, the user is referred to the following World Wide Web site for current information: www.med4th.com/BASIS/

APPENDIX E

TABLES FOR FREQUENTLY USED TESTS AND TREATMENTS

Frequently Used Treatments

Use this table to store parameters for treatments you frequently utilize.

Treatment	Side Effect Frequency	Side Effect Impact	Betterment Frequency	Betterment Impact	Action Threshold	Remarks

Action Threshold% = (Side effect Frequency × Impact)/(Betterment Frequency × Impact)

Frequently Used Tests

Use this table to store parameters for tests you frequently utilize.

Diagnosis	Prev.	Test	Sens	Spec	LR+	LR–	Remarks

Likelihood Ratio (LR) (+) = Sensitivity/(1 – Specificity)
Likelihood Ratio (LR) (–) = (1 – Sensitivity)/Specificity

Odds = Prob/(1 – Prob)
Prob = Odds/(1 + Odds)
PostOdds = PreOdds × Likelihood Ratio

REFERENCES

1. Sox HC, et al. Medical Decision Making. Stoneham, MA: Butterworth-Heineman;1988.

2. Komaroff AL, Pass TM, Aronson MD, et al. The prediction of streptococcal pharyngitis in adults. J Gen Intern Med. 1986;1-7.

3. Detsky AS, et al. Primer on medical decision analysis. Medical Decis Making. 1997;17(2):123-56.

4. Fletcher RH, et al. Clinical Epidemiology: The Essentials. 3rd ed. New York: Williams & Wilkins; 1996.

5. Williams JW Jr, Simel DL, Roberts L, et al. Clinical evaluation for sinusitis: making the diagnosis by history and physical examination. Ann Intern Med. 1992;117:705-10.

6. Cirrhosis of the Liver. Scientific American Medicine Online Edition. 1998;4(IX):9.

7. Infective endocarditis. Scientific American Medicine Online Edition. 1998;7(XVIII):2-3.

8. Pauker SC, Kassirer JP. The threshold approach to clinical decision making. N Engl J Med. 1980;302:1109-17.

9. Allison JE, Tekawa IS, Ransom LJ, Adrain AL. A comparison of fecal occult–blood tests for colorectal-cancer screening. N Engl J Med. 1996;334:155-9.

10. Panzer RJ, et al. Diagnostic Strategies for Common Medical Problems. Philadelphia: American College of Physicians;1991.

11. Lewis RF, Abrahamowicz M, Cote R, et al. Predictive power of duplex ultrasonography in asymptomatic carotid disease. Ann Intern Med. 1997;127:13-20.

12. Sauve JS, Laupacis A, Ostbye T, et al. Does this patient have a clinically important carotid bruit? JAMA. 1993;270:2843-5.

13. Lee TT, Solomon NA, Heidenreich PA, et al. Cost-effectiveness of screening for carotid artery testing: a meta-analytic review. Ann Intern Med. 1995;122:360-7.

14. Blakeley DD, Oddone EZ, Hasselblad V, et al. Noninvasive carotid artery testing: a meta-analytic review. Ann Intern Med. 1995;122:360-7.

15. Hobson RW II, Weiss DG, Fields WS, et al. Efficacy of carotid endarterectomy for asymptomatic carotid stenosis. N Engl J Med. 1993;328:221-7.

16. Sonnenberg FA. Decision analysis in disease management. Disease Management and Clinical Outcomes. 1997;1(1):20-34.

INDEX

⊰∙⊱

ABOUT THE AUTHOR

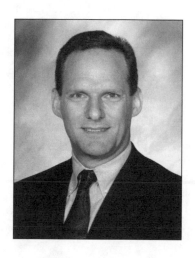

Richard Gross, MD, FACP, is Professor of Medicine in the Department of Medicine, Section of General Internal Medicine, at the University of Wisconsin Medical School. His experience includes fifteen years in private practice before entering academic medicine. In 1989 he designed and programmed a major electronic medical record program (Care4th®), later distributed commercially in 45 states. Since entering the world of academia, Dr. Gross has turned to evidence-based medicine and decision analysis in his teaching and programming efforts, incorporating many of the concepts of both disciplines into a major software project nearing completion. Caring for patients remains his preferred professional activity.